Reflexology
Massage

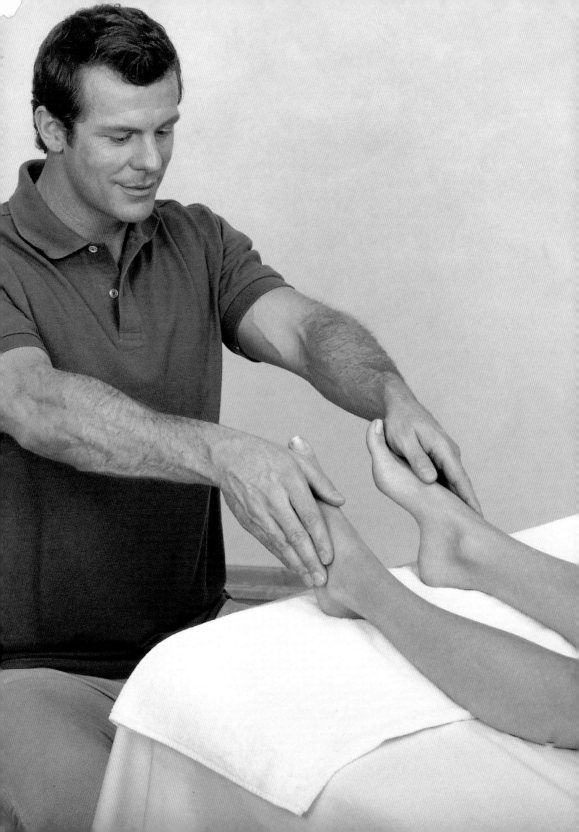

Monika Schaefer

Reflexology Massage

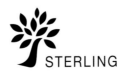

STERLING

New York / London
www.sterlingpublishing.com

Dedication
For Lena, Carla, and Eva

STERLING and the distinctive Sterling logo are
registered trademarks of Sterling Publishing Co., Inc.

Library of Congress Cataloging-in-Publication Data Available

10 9 8 7 6 5 4 3 2 1

Published by Sterling Publishing Co., Inc.
387 Park Avenue South, New York, NY 10016
Originally published under the title
Reflexzonenmassage © 2006 BLV Buchverlag GmbH & Co. KG, München/Germany
English translation ©2008 by Sterling Publishing Co., Inc.
Distributed in Canada by Sterling Publishing
c/o Canadian Manda Group, 165 Dufferin Street
Toronto, Ontario, Canada M6K 3H6
Distributed in the United Kingdom by GMC Distribution Services
Castle Place, 166 High Street, Lewes, East Sussex, England BN7 1XU
Distributed in Australia by Capricorn Link (Australia) Pty. Ltd.
P.O. Box 704, Windsor, NSW 2756, Australia

Sterling ISBN-13: 978-1-4027-4763-2
        ISBN-10: 1-4027-4763-2

For information about custom editions, special sales, premium and
corporate purchases, please contact Sterling Special Sales
Department at 800-805-5489 or specialsales@sterlingpublishing.com.

Liability Disclaimer
In this book, you will become familiar with foot reflexology as a simple and very effective method for physical and mental relaxation as well as for the vitalization and strengthening of your wellness-maintaining forces. For the treatment of existing ailments or illnesses, reflexology belongs in the hands of an experienced therapist. The information and advice given in this book have been carefully taken under consideration and examined by the author and the publication house. Nevertheless, no guarantees can be made. The author and the publication house as well as its employees cannot be held liable for personal, material, and property damage.

Contents

Preface

Bringing "Balance" to Body and Soul

This book is addressed to people who find pleasure in indulging in calm and relaxing time spent together, particularly in massaging the reflex zones of the feet and hands. Since reflexology is counted among the "ordering procedures," you will notice that such a massage can bring "order" to your partner and to yourself. By "order," I mean an inner peace that counters the daily stress that can often wreak havoc with our sense of balance. This applies equally to young and old, men and women, and those active professionally or those managing a family.

Massaging the hands and stimulating the reflex points located on the dorsum of the hand and palm can be very good alternatives to massaging the feet. Hands can be reached more easily than feet and so are perfectly suited for self-massage. Furthermore, they can be a great transition for those people who feel rather uncomfortable when it comes to somebody else touching their feet.

In the following pages, you will find and learn many reflexology techniques to foster relaxation, to strengthen the immune system, and to promote health. I cordially invite you to try out right away what you have read, to turn theory into practice, for there are many forms of establishing contact via hands and feet. Test your intuition and the fine-tuning of your senses as you massage. Proceed step by step as you might easily become overwhelmed if you try too many grips at once. In this way you will continue to find joy in massaging, and you will notice that you become increasingly confident after each treatment. It is important to mention that this book is not intended as a guide in the medical sense.

It is possible to treat many illnesses using reflexology massage, although "treatment" is defined solely as providing therapy. Considerations of care necessitate that reflex zone therapy as medical treatment may only be carried out by medically qualified personnel such as, for example, doctors, homeopaths, and (on doctor's orders) by physiotherapists and nursing personnel. Because I have written this book for the layperson, when I use terms like "treating" and "treatment," this should be understood to mean "doing something with your hands"—and not interpreted in the medical or judicial sense.

Have fun reading and experimenting!
Monika Schaefer

What Is Foot Reflexology?

Why, of All Parts, the Feet?

When you look down at yourself, you will notice that it is your feet that establish contact with the ground. Our feet carry us through life, even in the figurative sense. When you get the chance, focus for a moment on the way you move about, on the way you walk. We can walk with a spring or bounce, mince, creep, hop, run, hurry, or jog. "We walk through life," "we stand our ground," "something is an uphill climb." How we stand and how we walk obviously play a very important role in life: "To stand with both feet firmly on the ground" or "to float on air." Language frequently employs images of solidity or instability that are directly linked to our feet.

An infant, when exploring his closest surroundings—namely his or her own body—likes to put toes or even the entire foot into his or her mouth. Although this is usually seen as an exercise in coarse and fine motor skills, it is, at the same time, an exploration of self-discovery and sensory pleasure. Wheelchair-bound people who are unable to actively use their feet find that a careful positioning of the feet on the footrests is quite important, since contact via the feet to the ground affects the entire body even when sitting. And everyone knows that massaging the feet is always a sensual experience, so let us give them our full attention!

Characteristics of Reflexology

Characteristic starting points in reflexology are relaxation, stimulation, harmonization, support, and order. This ensures that the human being is supported in (re-)attaining inner and outer balance and then stabilizing it. Reflexology means putting down your hands, laying hands upon someone, touching others, and allowing yourself to be touched. It can have an effect on both the physical as well as the mental levels, and this is true not only when it is given by professional therapists, but also—and perhaps especially—when you massage a child, your partner, a friend, or a sick human being.

Setting Specific Stimuli

Massaging the foot's reflex zones can help you to feel the ground under your feet. In the following sections, you will learn how to stimulate the physical and mental levels via specific sets of actions.

Significance of the Hands: Touch and Movement

Stimulation is provided by your hands through pressure, stroking, or holding. Everyday contact, such as an embrace, holding hands, taking a child by the hand, shaking hands, or stroking someone to soothe or comfort, generally has a positive effect. You will become increasingly aware of the significance of your hands through foot reflexology. Touch and movement have a direct effect, but they also work inversely, for the action of the senses have a reciprocal effect: I cannot touch without being touched or move without being moved.

The Way Foot Reflexology Works

By now it is somewhat common knowledge that a connection exists between the reflex zones on the foot and the corresponding organs and systems in the body. Interactions become palpable for the person being massaged through sensations both on the foot—in the form of pleasant pricking, a warm sensation, tickling, or pressure pain—as well as in the body—as pressure relief, tickling, or a warm sensation.

It is generally claimed that the stimulus runs from the foot and is directed via nerve tracts to the corresponding area in the body. Although this is not correct, it is still useful as a model of thought. Some therapists talk of energy channels, while others compare the way reflexology works with that of the meridians in traditional Chinese medicine (TCM). Currently, how foot reflexology really works is not clear.

Based on experience with correctly applied massages, it can be said that the stimulation of certain pressure points on the foot leads to reactions within the associated organs and thus to a relaxation of the entire organism. Different reactions during massage, such as sensations of warmth or tickling, show that the mechanisms involved are not subject to the deliberate, cognizant regulation of and control through our cerebrum. They are instead assigned to our so-called autonomous nervous system, which consists of two parts, the sympathetic nerve and the parasympathetic nerve, and which reacts involuntarily. These as-of-now unknown mechanisms link certain zones of the foot with associated areas of the body.

Starting from the assumption that massage has many (inter-)connections that are as complex as the human organism itself, my own experience with this treatment is that therapists bring to the treatment the virtues of intuition, respect, and empathy, which have noticeably positive effects on the person receiving the massage. In other words, within us and within the other person, there exist invisible oscillations that we can make use of when we massage, thus making each treatment a unique experience.

■ There are interactions between the zones on the foot and the associated organs in the body.

Reactions can be noticed in foot and body. Foot reflexology has a balancing effect on body and soul.

When carrying out a reflexology treatment, one may observe an increased blood flow to the organ that shows a connection to the massaged zone on the foot. In a study done by the University Hospital for Internal Medicine in Innsbruck, Austria, it was demonstrated that with a correctly applied massage of the kidney zones, the blood flow of the kidney arteries improved significantly. Furthermore, observers noted effects on the autonomous nervous system in the form of relaxation, improved sleeping ability, as well as increased ease of excretion.

Historic Overview

In many cultures and ethnic groups, massaging the feet has significant meaning. From ancient Egypt more than 4,000 years ago, we find images of the art of healing on or through the feet. Because these images come from a tomb, we can speculate that the deceased earned his living with this activity. In India and China, foot therapy was likewise practiced. Around the time when acupuncture was established in China, the massage of certain pressure points of the feet became a recognized form of healing.

At the beginning of the twentieth century, the American physician, Dr. William Fitzgerald (1872-1942), began to explore Indian and Chinese folk medicine. As an ear, nose, and throat doctor, he had served at various hospitals in Boston, London, and Vienna. He observed that physical organ functioning could be influenced by targeted massage and explored this phenomenon in his 1917 work *Zone Therapy*. With the partitioning of the body into different zones (see p. 10), he laid the foundation for today's foot reflexology and, with his colleague Dr. Joe S. Riley, later developed the subject further.

▼

Even this recumbent Buddha shows something like "reflex zones" on his soles.

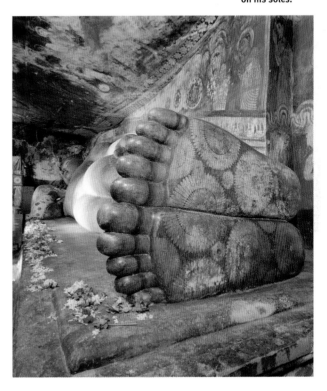

However, it was Eunice D. Ingham, a Canadian physical therapist, who pressed ahead with the practical work. She concentrated her massage work on the zones of the feet and not, as Fitzgerald had done, on body zones in general. In this way, she delved more and more deeply into the realm of foot reflex zones, the experience of which she published as a book entitled *Stories the Feet Can Tell*. Soon thereafter, a second publication followed called *Stories the Feet Have Told*. Through these studies, foot reflexology was introduced to an increasingly wider public.

In Germany in the 1960s, Hanne Marquardt, having discovered Ingham's books, also recognized the "key functioning of the feet" in her own physiotherapeutic practice as it first had been described by Ingham: "from which, I did not

▼
Fitzgerald partitioned the body into two times five vertical zones as well as into four horizontal levels.

know how and why, effects could be triggered in the entire body!" After meeting Eunice Ingham in person, she made it her life's work to establish foot reflexology in Germany.

In the United States, England, and Scandinavian countries, therapy via the feet is used as a preventative and medical therapy. It is also accepted and used as a simple and effective home remedy.

A Little Bit of Theory . . .

In order to enable you to work independently on the feet and to make you comfortable in dealing with the reflex zones, I will now introduce two theoretical principles of foot reflexology. Feel free to use it as a "cheat sheet" during a massage.

Zone Partitioning According to Fitzgerald

First, you should become familiar with Dr. W. Fitzgerald's zone partitioning. In his 1917 work *Zone Therapy*, Fitzgerald focuses mainly on various massage devices that he had developed; here, you will also find the illustration of the body with the often-cited zone therapy chart.

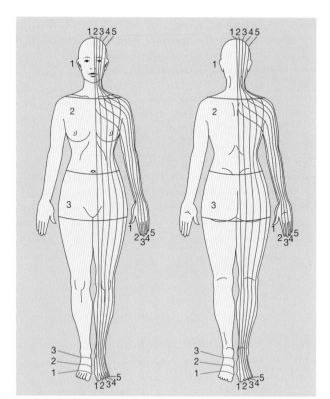

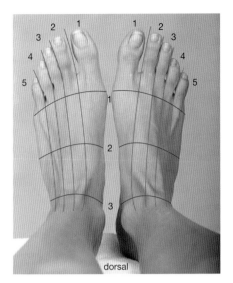

dorsal

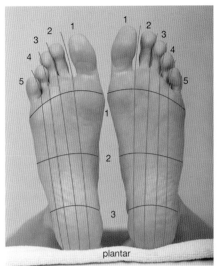

plantar

Left:
Partitioning of zones according to Fitzgerald; analogous zones on the tops of the feet (dorsum).

Right:
Analogous zones on the soles of the feet (plantar).

Fitzgerald divided the human body vertically into two sets of five zones running parallel through the body extending from the head to the feet and toes. Zone 1, positioned in the middle, is equally valid for both the right and the left half of the body; in the extremities, it then appears once right and once left. This is significant for the foot massage referring to those organs located in the center of the body. Later, Fitzgerald added three horizontal lines. You will encounter these levels again later as "regions" in the practical part, "Foot Reflexology—Zones and Organs" beginning on page 49.

Fitzgerald theorized that it might very well be possible to influence each organ located within a certain vertical zone from other points along the vertical zone by means of massage or various massage devices that he had developed.

The horizontal levels within the zone chart of the human body gained in significance only later, after students and colleagues of Fitzgerald and especially Eunice D. Ingham, who was instrumental in this matter, had moved the feet into the foreground.

The horizontal levels stand for:
1. The area of the head and shoulders
2. The chest and upper abdomen
3. The lower abdomen and the area of the pelvis, including the legs

Correspondingly, the horizontal levels can be found on the foot.

Example:
■ The human intestines are located in the area of the abdomen where they are stretched out across the entire width as small and large intestines.

■ In the zone partitioning according to Fitzgerald, each is located in the area of the vertical body zones 1 to 5, right and left, and in the area of the upper part of the third horizontal level.

■ Thus, in terms of the foot, the intestine area can be massaged both right and left across the entire width of both feet since the vertical zones run all the way down. The horizontal levels likewise correspond to their respective regions.

■ Since it makes sense to massage the reflex zones of the intestine on the sole of the foot (the dorsum of the foot is very bony in this area), you will find them in the lower area of the sole of the foot just above the heel (see the practical part beginning on p. 49).

The reflex zones on the hands follow similar rules of correspondence. However, it has been shown that the treatment of the feet has a more intense effect on the organs and the quality of relaxation runs deeper. Still, you will find several suggestions regarding massaging the hands and their reflex zones in the practical section beginning on page 85.

▶
From a side view, the foot resembles a sitting man. If you change your viewpoint a little—to get a "tilt picture"—you will be able to see that resemblence.

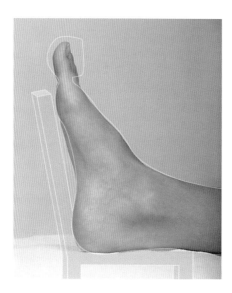

Form Analogy According to Marquardt

The assigned reflex zones on the dorsum and the sole of the foot correspond to the order of the body, to its organs and its functions. The objective is to see both an erect foot and a sitting person simultaneously. Hanne Marquardt illustrated this in her book *Reflexzonentherapie am Fuß* (*Foot Reflexology*): a foot whose profile, when seen perpendicular to the surface, is reminiscent of a sitting person. This is comparable to the famous "tilt pictures," where one image or another—depending on the vantage point—appears before one's eyes.

■ For practical reasons, it is useful to play around with similarities of shape: "Tilt" the images in several directions. Such prominent points as head, back, spine, chest, pelvis/posterior are very helpful as signposts in this respect.

So, jot down the analogy of foot and body on your imaginary "cheat sheet." Seeing the physical shape of the foot as an analogy of the body in conjunction with Fitzgerald's zone partitioning will allow you to become more secure in your dealings with the reflex zones as you work.

The Zone Chart

On pages 14 and 15, you will find an overview of all foot reflex zones that are discussed in this book.

At first sight, this might seem rather daunting. Take it as an "overview" in the literal sense of the word: a bird's-eye view of how complex foot reflex zone work truly is. Besides, you cannot expect to know everything right away; after all, you are just starting out on your journey.

> You will find basic tips for applying foot reflexology in this chapter from page 16 on, as well as in the chapter "Grips and Techniques That You Should Be Familiar With," beginning on page 28.

When You Should Not Give a Massage

Foot reflexology works with energies that are already present in the body. For this reason, you, as a layperson, should proceed with caution in any situation in which the physical or mental balance of the person receiving the massage is disturbed. For example:

■ When a person has an infectious disease or feverish infection (for example, flu, infections, or children's diseases), you should not massage.

■ If a person has an increased tendency to bleed or illnesses of the blood vessels, you should likewise forgo pressure point massage.

■ In situations where your "experimentee" is suffering from cramps, avoid the activation of stimuli in the area of the head zones on the feet (see pp. 52–57).

You may, however, always use the stroke movements explained in the chapter "Grips and Techniques That You Should Be Familiar With" (beginning on p. 28), the positioning of your hands under the heel, or the "laying on" of your hand. With these movements, you are not initiating an active stimulus but rather soothing what is afflicted, and, in addition, you are strengthening the other person's immune system. You may also just simply hold your thumb, index finger, or the palm of your hand on the reflex zone that is assigned to the organ affected.

Keep in mind that sick children and the elderly also enjoy this kind of attention!

> Do not perform massages of the reflex zones with certain illnesses.
> Among these are:
> • Infections accompanied by fever
> • Fungus on the foot (thin cotton socks should be worn)
> • Mental illnesses with multiple symptoms (e.g., schizophrenia)
> • Suspicion of thrombosis
> • Suspicion of seizure
> • Acute inflammations in the vein or lymph systems

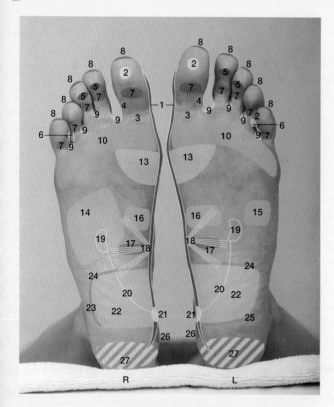

Overview of the reflex zones on the soles
of the feet:
1. Spine
2. Pituitary gland
3. Thyroid gland
4. Palatal tonsil
5. Eyes
6. Ears
7. Teeth
8. Sinusitis
9. Lymph in the head area
10. Shoulder region
13. Heart
14. Liver/gallbladder
15. Spleen
16. Stomach
17. Pancreas
18. Solar plexus
19. Kidneys
20. Urethra
21. Urinary bladder
22. Small intestine
23. Ascendant colon
24. Horizontal colon
25. Descendant colon
26. Anus
27. Pelvic floor

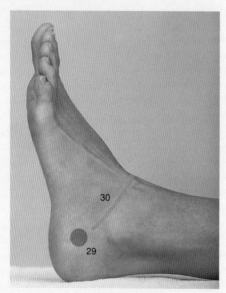

Overview of the reflex zones on the outer side
of the foot (mirrored on other foot):
29. Ovary/penis/testicles
30. Fallopian tube/spermatic duct/lymph
    in the groin area

▶

Overview of the reflex zones on the dorsum of the feet:
1. Spine
7. Teeth
11. Lungs/bronchae
12. Shoulder joint and upper arm
30. Fallopian tube/spermatic duct/lymph in the groin area

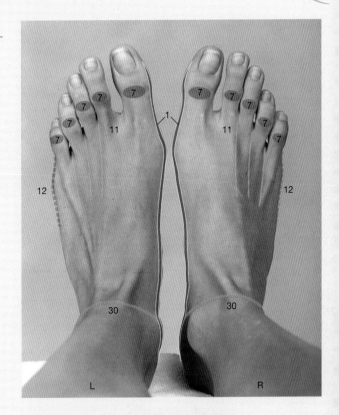

▶

Overview of the reflex zones on the inner side of the foot (mirrored on other foot):
1a. Cervical spine
1b. Thoracic spine
1c. Lumbar spine
1d. Sacrum
1e. Tailbone
28. Uterus/prostate
30. Fallopian tube/spermatic duct/lymph in the groin area

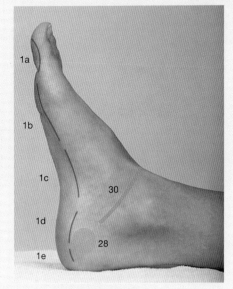

►
 Be patient with yourself as you learn the massage!

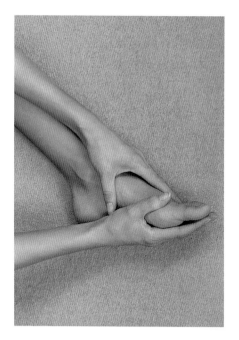

Tips for Successfully Learning Massage

In the following pages, you will be exposed to a great deal of new information. The idea of having foot reflex zones will open up an entirely new world for you and give you a new-found appreciation of your feet! There are many possibilities to approach this subject. Read through the following suggestions, and then decide which is the best for you.

From the Beginning to the End

Pick up the book and merely read it from the beginning to the end. Then, try out the suggestions for the practical exercises.

Some Theory and Right into the Practice

Read through the first three theoretical chapters. Then review the information regarding "Preparations for the Massage" (p. 17). Next, I recommend "General Information Regarding Foot Reflexology" (p. 42), followed by "Grips and Techniques That You Should Be Familiar With" (p. 28). Then begin your practical applications with the stroke movements presented.

Step by Step—Your Back First

One strategy is to begin with energy-stroking (p. 34). Next, you massage the inner edge of the feet (which corresponds, as a reflex zone, to the back) and progress to the toes (the reflex zone of the head region). Then you wrap up the massage with yet another energy stroke. During your next massage, you will add another section, and you will continue in this way until you have massaged the entire foot over the course of several sessions. (You will find the description of the individual reflex zones beginning on p. 49.)

Do You Want to Start Right Away?

Then I recommend the section "Stroking and Balancing Techniques" beginning on page 34. Here you can read up on the energy stroke, which is a great way to begin the massage.

▋ Be patient with yourself no matter which approach to learning you decide on!

Preparations for the Massage

How to Prepare Yourself

Your own preparation for the massage begins with becoming attuned to your inner self and to the task at hand. This means that you should make the time to concentrate solely on the massage and to be awake and attentive to the subtle reactions of your partner.

This does not require special abilities but rather only practice, especially practice in readying your outer temporal and inner concentrated free time for the next half hour.

Preparing Your Environment

It likewise makes sense to prepare the immediate environment where you will be performing the massage. It does not take much: radio, TV equipment, and CD-player should be switched off and your telephone or cell phone should be placed in another room. If you like, you can listen to relaxing music; however, I recommend that you let the relaxation come from the silence and the massage work itself.

Find out how sonorous silence can be.

Inner Peace and Outer Silence as a Preparation for the Massage

Ask yourself, do I take my own inner and outer preparation for the massage seriously? If this is the case, then you are setting the course for a successful treatment that will grant well-being and relaxation. What a wonderful gift it can be to devote time and attention to yourself and to your partner!

▼

A quiet environment lends itself to a great massage.

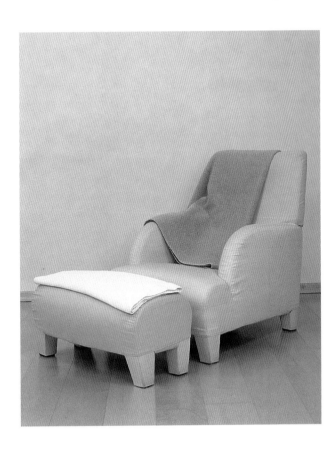

Giving and Receiving— Two Important Elements

At the beginning of my training as a foot reflexology therapist, I was glad to have my children as receptive (and patient!) test subjects. They gave me some excellent constructive criticism during our sessions. The children enjoyed feeling the sequence of various grips, which, though initially insecure and searching, became, with time, more and more experienced.

In this way, I found that receiving foot reflexology was not the only delight; carrying it out brought just as much joy. To experience the trust given, to feel the effects of the reflexology therapy that you are giving, and to see how you facilitate relaxation with your hands—all this can be very gratifying.

> Despite the delight that comes with a massage, you should not do it if you feel sick or overtired.

Possible Reasons for Foot Reflexology

Foot reflexology is always useful when the physical or mental forces are out of balance, or simply—as when we go to a sauna—to indulge in something good.

Possible reasons for such a treatment can be:
- Aches (e.g., back-, head-, or stomach aches)
- Digestive problems (constipation)
- Sleeping problems
- "Inner unrest"
- With school children before a test
- Disposition to high blood pressure
- Menstrual discomfort
- Discomfort during menopause
- Convalescence
- Care of the seriously ill and dying

Frequency of Massages

If you would like to massage someone regularly, one or two massages per week are advisable. After 10 treatments, you can have a longer break of six to eight weeks. During this time, the stimuli continue to take effect in the body.

> Stimuli set within the framework of the massage should alternate with breaks so that the body's own reactions can unfold.

Optimal Timing

Decide on a time to meet with a close friend on the weekend or on a free evening and massage one another.

It is important that you both are willing to invest an hour of your time and not mentally rush ahead to your next activity!

With smaller children, I recommend the times just before or after their nap. With school children, evening and just before bedtime are good opportunities for massage.

A Suitable Place

The location for the massage should be chosen in such a way that the person receiving the massage lies comfortably on his or her back and you are sitting in a relaxed manner. You may use the living room sofa, a bed, or you may even place several blankets or a mat on the floor. If you choose the floor, you may find that a shiatsu mat is the most comfortable. It is well cushioned and large enough that you can even find room for yourself at the end of the mat.

You must also find a comfortable position for yourself. Even a comfortable, reclining garden chair can be used. Whatever you decide on, make sure that it supports your back and that your knees are comfortable and not stressed or strained. If you can manage to sit for a long time cross-legged, then the floor or the end of a sofa

or bed will not be a problem for you. However, if this is not the case, you may also use an extendable table cushioned with blankets as an improvised massage table. Be inventive and try out several possibilities. It is very important that the person giving the massage has a good seating position. Tension caused by an uncomfortable posture lessens the pleasure given by the massage and can affect the entire treatment.

Your Posture

Since access to professional equipment is limited in the home environment (e.g., only a sofa or bed may be available), a certain flexibility in terms of your own posture is required.

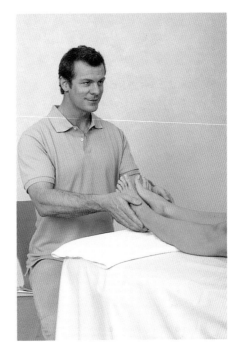

If the person receiving the massage is lying on a bed or a chaise, position yourself at its end on a chair or stool so that you can easily reach the feet with your hands. Your feet should have firm contact with the ground.

Sitting Positions

● Does the bed or sofa have a raised armrest or footboard at the end where the feet are? If so, I recommend that you work cross-legged. Alternatively, you can bend one leg and place the other one on the floor. Be sure to change your position before the joints hurt too much.

● If the bed or the chaise has no obstruction at the feet but it is too low for you to comfortably sit on a chair in front of it, then you should use a small stool or footstool.

● What if you are massaging on the floor? You should alternate between sitting cross-legged and "heel sitting" (bending the knees and sitting on your heels). Or you can try kneeling on one knee and resting the other foot on the floor. It is important to move, though, so that your legs do not fall asleep.

Seating Possibilities

● Are you sitting comfortably? Can you rest your feet on the floor while having a firm grip? It is important to have a good contact with the floor!

● You should be able to easily move your chair or stool during the massage. Depending on which area of the foot you are working, a change in your sitting position can be useful.

● A softer seat can let you sink in and can subsequently prevent you from maintaining good posture. On the other hand, a hard seat can soon hurt your posterior. Something in the middle, like a bolstered chair, may feel the most comfortable.

▶

If sitting on your heels for an extended period of time does not cause discomfort, then this is a well-suited massage position. However, change the position before it becomes uncomfortable.

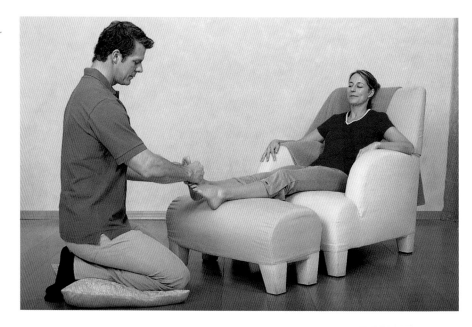

Positioning of Foot and Leg

Place your feet and legs about hip width apart; they should be even and relaxed, not too wide, too narrow, or crossed. It may help to think of hip width as being the same as shoulder width. With this posture, you can place both feet firmly on the ground, so that you are well grounded and rooted.

While massaging, you should check the position of your feet every so often. Perhaps you are only touching the ground with the tip of your foot, or maybe your knees are pulled upward? Your shoulders may be raised as well, and your breathing may be strained. One after the other, release the outer tensions, and the inner ones should follow. Then your breathing will come more naturally.

> Try to walk barefoot in the summer or only wear socks at home. In doing so, your awareness of your own feet and their contact to the ground will intensify.

Posture of Posterior and Pelvis

Your posterior should have good contact with your chair seat. Keep the pelvis properly aligned: the hips should be neither tilted backward nor bent forward. Can you feel your thighs as a connection between your pelvis and your knees? These body parts, followed by your lower legs and the ankle joints, connect to your feet.

Feel your own body. Feel how you are seated! It is important to pay attention to the tone of your own body. Sitting tensed on the front edge of your chair or leaning back against the back of your chair are both unbalanced ways of approaching the massage.

> "Posture and gesture express what lives inside, what our heart feels, and express our senses—but they also affect our inner being, give it strength, shape and educate it . . ."
> *Romano Guardini*

The Posture of the Back and Spine

Try to straighten up at first from the inside and then from the outside as well, starting from your pelvis via the lumbar spine, the thoracic spine, the cervical spine, and the back of the head up to the crown. Have you ever heard of the imaginary thread that, starting from the back of your head or rather your spine, pulls you upward toward the sky? Use this image to straighten your spine. With the correct posture, your inner organs gain the space that they need. When the lobes of the lungs have space, you are able to breathe in deeply and fully. You may even want to let loose a big sigh that comes from deep within. Now there is enough room to do so!

Furthermore, with the correct posture, your intestines are not squeezed and can relax along the entire length of more than 23 feet (7 meters). Also, the heavily branched nervous system in the area of the stomach, the so-called solar plexus, can stretch even the smallest extensions of the nerve endings.

When you straighten your upper body so that you can breathe deeply, you will instinctively roll your shoulders back and down creating further relaxation.

All of this enables comfortable posture with good body tone. Combined with a little bit of stretching exercises, you may even be surprised by how tall you really are!

Positioning of Arms and Hands

Rely on gravity, and simply let your arms drop. Upper arm, elbow, forearm, wrist, hand, and fingers, everything is linked with one another and forms a whole with the extremity that starts at the shoulder joint. Now bend your forearms to a right angle in the elbow joint—this is more or less your work posture. The pep and vigor of your massage comes ultimately from your stable seating position and is relayed via spine and shoulders, upper- and lower arms to your hands with massaging thumb and index finger.

> Your posture stabilizes your body; the relationship of body tone and the feeling carried via feet, posterior, and spine has a decisive influence on the dynamic of the massage.

Positioning the Head

See if you notice tension in the neck and jaw area and in the cervical spine when you sit upright. Your posture should be alert but loose. While applying the massage, every so often take the time to look away, for example, out a window; you will notice that the thumb and index finger will do their work and that you can follow the treatment much better with your inner eye than with your outer eyes. Many of my participants report that they work much better when they do not look at the feet or their massaging hands.

Distance to the Feet

The distance between you and the feet to be massaged should be enough so that you can easily reach them with a right-angled forearm. Pay attention that you neither get too close to the person nor allow the distance between you to become too great. If the person being massaged is lying on a chaise or a bed, his or her feet should be perpendicular to and even with the foot of the bed.

The Most Frequent Mistakes in Posture

At the beginning, you will unconsciously tend to adjust the distance to the foot by repositioning your upper body and/or posterior. It often happens that the upper body is bent so far forward that the tip of your nose seems to almost touch the big toe. Or the posterior slips all the way to the front edge of the chair, your heels are pulled up, and the tips of your toes are tense.

To correct this, keep your shoulders back and tuck your chin keeping your head comfortably balanced over your shoulders. Although these are the most common mistakes, there are many others that can occur.

Relaxed and Concentrated Working

■ Pay attention to your posture as you continue to massage or as you keep your hands on the feet. Re-assert tone where it becomes lost, and loosen those body parts that have become strained.

■ Relax from the feet upward via the lower legs and the knees (the hollows of the knees are often tensed unconsciously) and continue through the thighs to the posterior and the pelvis. How are you sitting now?

■ What follows next is the straightening of your spine all the way up to your imaginary thread (see p. 21).

■ Now give your chest some attention. Does it only open up for a deep breath?

■ Finally, bring your shoulders, arms, fingers, and thumbs into a correct working position (see preceding paragraphs). And on we go with our massage!

Sharpened Perception

Do not, under any circumstances, skimp on the time intended for preparing yourself, for practicing and feeling your way into a correct sitting position, and for perceiving your own body's state. The more attentive you are to yourself, the more alert you will become to the verbal and nonverbal signals that are sent out by your partner. You will not miss the loosely positioned feet or the slightly tensed heels pressed into the pad, and so you will be able to react with circumspection and consideration.

Warm Hands and Feet—For You As Well

Be very sure that you have warm feet and hands!

For people with chronically cold hands—or feet—I recommend that they indulge in a warm foot or hand bath. Submerge your feet to just above the ankle, and your hands can sink in well beyond the elbows. You will be surprised at how pleasant this is. If your hands do not stay warm, you could purchase a warming pad of the size of your palm made of synthetic material. It contains a bendable metal plate that crystallizes the liquid inside. Use this to warm your hands first, and then place the pad under you (if you squeeze it once in a while, it will stay warm longer). If your hands cool off again, then the pad is right there to use once more.

Generally, however, your hands will take on a pleasant work temperature in the course of the reflexology.

Other Things to Consider

- Wear comfortable clothes when you offer a massage. Avoid pants that are too tight—you will only feel constrained, especially if, for example, you have pulled your legs into a cross-legged position.
- You should also take off any jewelry, such as bracelets or rings. These can be unpleasant on the feet, and they can also disturb you. Wedding bands are all right, though, since most are flat and unobtrusive.
- Leave the wristwatch behind, since both you and your partner "tick" differently than a battery-operated watch. You will notice in your pulse or breathing that you have a very different rhythm than your timepiece.
- Given the circumstances, your fingernails should be kept rather short. Of course, while you may keep your nails longer, doing so will cause you to have to position your thumb in a slightly more leveled fashion (see p. 28). When you look at your fingers or thumb from behind, the respective nail should not be visible, if possible.
- Overall, your movements should be calm. Now, the nice thing is that this happens almost automatically while massaging. With my seminars, I regularly enjoy the pleasant, quiet, yet concentrated atmosphere that comes with participants giving one another massages.

Getting into the Right Massage Mood

The Footbath

In order to get into the foot reflexology mood, a warm footbath that reaches above the ankles is relaxing and cathartic for body and soul. Even when you massage yourself, take this time (see p. 76) and enjoy the relaxing effect of the water. If, though, the person opposite you is already lying down and you immediately notice that he or she has very cold feet, then I recommend a "horizontal footbath."

For this, you will need two towels. Wet one of them in running hot water, and place the other one nearby. Firmly wring out the wet towel, and leave it gathered together. Unfold it just before you use it, and check the temperature with the back of your hand. Hold it against the soles of the feet, and wrap it around the toes and outer ankles. Since the warmth in the towel dissipates very quickly, using your hands, press the towel against the feet for a moment. Afterward, dry the feet with the nearby towel, and cover the feet while you take away the used towels. A "horizontal footbath" is effective and very pleasant. You may want to try it out!

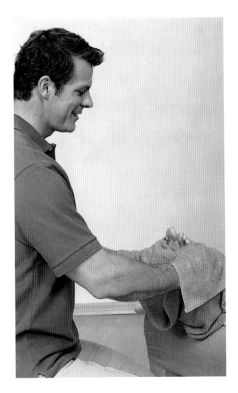

With hot, damp towels you will get your partner's feet to the ideal "operating temperature."

Positioning

Before starting the massage, first pay attention to your sitting position, and then move on to the person opposite you. Is he or she lying comfortably? Remember that this person should be able to spend a solid half-hour on his or her back.

Offer the person a knee roll, small pillow, or a rolled-up blanket. Is the head comfortable, or would a higher or flatter pillow be better? If the person has back problems, a small pillow or a folded towel placed under the backs of the knees or the small of the back can have a miraculous effect. Be sure to ask and to offer alternatives! Most people will answer the question whether they are lying comfortably with "Yes, thank you. It works," only to find out that a small pillow placed in the right spot can optimize the position.

Covering

Some people find being covered burdensome or constricting. Nonetheless, a blanket is useful because the body will cool off slightly during the massage. In summer, you may want to use a light bed sheet. Careful covering provides a feeling of security: "I am warmly embraced, and now things can begin."

This entire preparation for the massage, from the choice of location, your own preparation, to the positioning of the person to be massaged, may initially appear elaborate and even unnecessary. However, if you make it a habit to invest time and effort in the preparation of the massage, you will quickly notice how it increases the overall quality.

Think of sewing clothing or applying wallpaper: The preparation always takes a lot of time. The same can be said of reflexology!

Orientation to the Hands and Feet

In order to get your bearings with regard to the hands and feet, some useful and objective definitions are explained in the following alphabetical listing. Feel free to add your own notes if you think that one term or another is lacking.

Term	Definition
Across:	Metatarsal arch describes the area below the toes along the front edge of the ball of the foot. It is the separating line between first and second levels according to Fitzgerald.
Arch:	This is the raised part of the sole of the foot that is usually not visible on a footprint.
Ball:	This is the part of the foot directly below the big toe. It has a raised and round shape; with adults, it often has calluses. When looking at a footprint, it is the widest part of the foot. For your practical work, divide the ball mentally into three parts: • Upper: directly below the big toe • Middle: the part that is arched forward between the upper and lower part • Bottom: connects with the middle section and runs downward toward the arch of the foot
Bottom:	This signifies the direction toward the heel.
Crown:	Observe your bare foot or hand: You will recognize the crowns on your toes and fingers where the fine lines of the friction ridges (your finger-prints) create the center point in your skin.
Distal joint:	Seen from the hand or the foot, it is located at the end of a finger or toe.
Dorsum of the foot:	Looking down at your feet you see the dorsum (top) of the foot.
Dorsum of the hand:	Putting your hands down in front of you, both thumbs on the inside, you see the dorsum (back) of your hand.
Edge of heel:	This is the boundary between the heel and the arch of the foot. It is also along the sides and to the back.
Heel:	This is the back section of a footprint (imagine a print in the sand or a wet foot on dry ground). It includes the part of the foot that rests on the surface when you lie on your back. It is also easily recognizable in sport socks since the heel is often reinforced or of a different color.
Inner edge:	This runs between the big toe and the heel.
Inside:	This indicates the direction toward the center of the body.

Levels:	W. H. Fitzgerald divides the body into four levels that correspond to the foot. In practice, we speak of "regions."
Longitudinal arch:	This is the arch when seen lengthwise from toe to heel.
Metacarpo-phalangeal joint:	This is the joint that establishes the connection between the fingers and hand or the toes and foot.
Metacarpo-phalangeal toe joint:	See "Metacarpophalangeal joint."
Outer edge:	This is the edge between the little toe and the heel.
Outside:	In terms of the foot, "outside" means everything that runs on the outer side of the foot or points in this direction.
Pad of index finger:	See "thumb pad."
Palm:	Turning your hands over, with the thumbs pointing outward, you look into the palm of your hand.
Pressure point massage:	Foot reflexology works through stimuli that are sent via the massage of certain reflex zones. The thumb or index finger exerts pressure (reflex point after reflex point).
Region:	This is what we call the various sections on the foot. Based on the division into regions, this structuring and orientation makes foot reflexology much easier.
Sole of the foot:	This part touches the floor as we walk. It has very sensitive tissue that is responsive to touch and temperature.
Tarso-metatarsal:	Here, we are dealing with the very difficult to access ends of the metatarsal bones; a small gap at the connecting point to the tarsal bones. According to Fitzgerald, these correspond with the zones between the second and the third levels.
Thumb pad:	Place your thumb on the edge of the tabletop, and rotate it to be perpendicular to the surface (the nail should not touch the table). Now you will be able to exert pressure onto the tabletop with your pad—this is how you apply the stimuli on the foot.
Tip of toe:	This is the area at the end of the toe, above the toenail.
Tissue:	The tissue of the skin is divided into the upper layer (or epidermis), the inner layer (dermis), and fat tissue. Within the various layers, there are tactile corpuscles, blood vessels, and nerve endings.
Top:	This signifies the direction toward the toes.
Zone:	This is an area on the foot that, as a reflex zone, corresponds to a certain part of the body and is thus assigned to it.

Grips and Techniques That You Should Be Familiar With

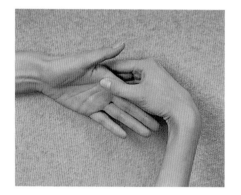

▶
The resting phase—the thumb is positioned.

The bulk of foot reflexology is carried out with the thumb, though the index and middle fingers are often involved. Stroke movements should be done with your flat hand.

Using the Thumb

Your thumb works its way forward in two phases that are rhythmically tuned to one another.

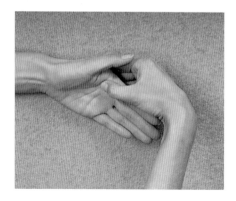

▶
The working phase—the thumb pad is pressed into the tissue.

■ First is the resting phase: Position the thumb on the tissue of the foot (for practice, use your hand). Pause there for a split second.
■ Second is the work phase: Press the pad of the thumb with appropriate enthusiasm into the tissue.

> The pressure does not come from the strength of the thumb but starts as a movement up in the shoulder and is carried through the upper arm, elbow, forearm, and hand into the thumb. Also, your inner attitude when massaging should be shaped by enthusiasm.

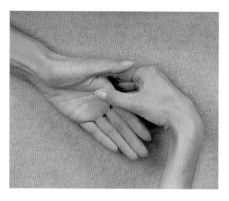

▶
In the following resting phase, the thumb glides with enthusiasm forward to the next point.

■ Then pause briefly with your thumb pad pressed into the tissue.

■ Now slowly release your thumb; then another resting phase follows.

■ How do you get to the next point? Although you have released your thumb slowly from the tissue of the foot, the work phase contains enough energy to carry out the entire movement (see above). This energy is sufficient to allow the thumb to glide forward at the end of the resting phase.

■ The next work phase then begins: Position the thumb, bringing the distal joint of the thumb perpendicular to the surface, and actively press the thumb in a vertical direction into the tissue of the foot.

■ This forward motion at the end of the resting phase and the glide into the next work phase happens almost automatically in the course of time. Do not push or press the thumb to the next point!

The alternation of the resting and work phases are reminiscent of the up and down of walking, of the in and out of breathing. See all of these as rhythmic sequences.

■ Be sure that your thumb is not led by the hand, trailing or dragged in a tilted position; the pad always applies the necessary pressure in a vertical direction from top to bottom, and the movement always runs forward. This means the thumb goes first, followed by the hand.

■ Picturing an ice skater might serve as a useful comparison. From the momentum of pushing off (the thumb moves energetically into the tissue), the skater glides for a while over the ice (resting phase as you move ahead to the next point), until next pushing off again using the momentum for yet another time (next work phase).

■ The significance of your posture, as described on page 19, will find its practical application at this point. I will elaborate on the resulting dynamic at the end of this chapter (see p. 47). Frequently with first massages, the pressure administered is too weak rather than too strong. You are best off asking your partner whether the pressure is right. The first spontaneous response will give you guidance for the remaining treatment.

Hand Massage—How to Practice the Use of the Thumb

Now put the parts just studied to work by first using your own hands as a training area. While this is not an explicit reflexology of the hand—you will become familiar with this starting on page 85—it is a valuable exercise for massaging individual reflex points with the thumb.

Preparation

Get comfortable for this exercise. You may use a small pillow so that the hand that you are about to massage has some support and can be positioned well. Later on, you will pay as much attention in positioning your partner!

Now, first observe your own hands: the dorsum of your hand, your palm, your fingers—your hands that grab, hold, stroke, or can be made into a fist.

Carrying Out Your Test Massage

■ Place your left hand into your right, and look into the left palm. The right thumb can now begin its work. Positioned on the so-called saddle joint, it is in the position to move in various directions and to stand opposite the other fingers.

■ With the right hand, support your left and begin the interplay of the resting and work phases. Get your right thumb moving; for the sake of simplicity, you may want to start on the left pad of the thumb. Massage the thumb on its inner side downward into the hand. Stop at the basal joint of the left thumb.

■ Next work on each finger progressing from the index to the little finger.

■ Finally, address the palm of the hand using horizontal lines. For this, position the thumb perpendicular to the surface on the distal joint, and press it into the tissue with a firm, yet flexible enthusiasm, pause a moment, release it, glide forward a fraction of an inch (a few millimeters), dive once again with enthusiasm into the depth while positioning the thumb perpendicular to the surface, pause once again, release the pressure, glide on. It is precisely at that moment in which you pause that the stimulus triggers the respective reflex point.

■ Try to carry out the resting and work phases in synchronization with your breathing rhythm. While breathing in, the thumb glides forward, and while breathing out it lowers into the depth. Pay attention to any change in your breathing rhythm and depth.

Completing the Practice Massage

■ As a finishing touch, you can stroke the left hand with your right. For this, put down the left hand (on the pillow) with the dorsum of your hand facing down, and stroke it with your right hand three times over a wide area from the wrist to the fingertips and beyond. Turn your hand over, and repeat the same stroking over the dorsum of your hand. You can also do this concurrent to your breathing rhythm. Are there changes? Do you sense the stroking more intensely?

■ When you are done, allow the left hand to rest for a little while on the pillow, and take a moment to take in how you feel after this little test massage. This resting period corresponds to the after-rest that follows the reflexology treatment (see p. 75).

■ Now switch hands and repeat the exercise.

Take your time with these self-exercises! Indulge in the stroking movements, and get a feeling for the right pressure and the thumb grip sequences.

Using the Index Finger

You may use your index finger—just as you can use the middle finger—as an alternative to the thumb. This will be necessary with certain reflex points on the dorsum of the foot (see also p. 57).

Likewise, you will often use the index finger concurrently with the thumb when you use the "claw-grip" shown on page 32.

The Index Finger Grip

■ As with the thumb, the index finger positions itself in the resting phase, perpendicular to the surface in its first finger joint.

■ Afterwards, it deepens with the energy from the shoulder, upper arm, elbow, forearm, and wrist into a reflex point, where it exerts pressure, pauses for a moment, releases itself again, and then glides forward to the next point.

Massaging the Dorsum of the Hand—How to Practice the Use of the Index Finger

Try the index finger grip on the dorsum of your hand.

■ Hold your left hand in front of you so that you look at the dorsum.

■ With the right index finger, slowly work your way into the "hollow" between the bones of the index and the middle finger all the way to the wrist.

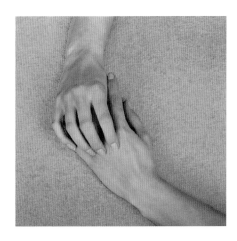

◄ The resting phase: The index finger is placed into position.

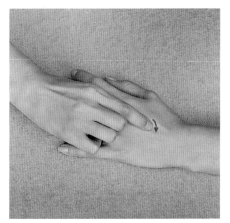

◄ The working phase: The index finger straightens and presses into the tissue.

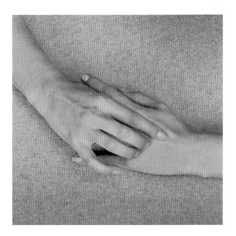

◄ The resting phase: The index finger glides forward to the next point. Another work phase follows.

▪ Massage the remaining two longitudinal valleys accordingly. Again, end with a stroking of the dorsum of your hand.

▪ Change your massaging and massaged hands so that the left index finger can now practice. Continue to think of the skater's momentum gliding over the ice. As you try out the index finger grip, concentrate on your own posture as well as on the hand to be massaged, which should be relaxed and positioned comfortably.

▪ Since people often hold their breath unconsciously when they concentrate, pay close attention that you are breathing calmly.

The Pinching Technique

With the pinching technique, the thumb and index finger exert pressure at the same time.

▼
Positioning of thumb and index finger with the pinching technique.

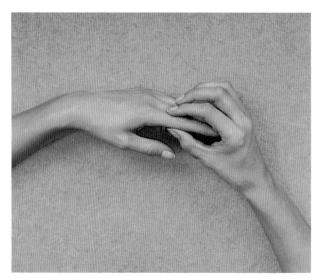

Finger Massage—How to Practice the Pinching Technique

▪ Once again, position the relaxed left hand in your lap or on a pillow with the dorsum facing upward. Now you work simultaneously with your right thumb and your index finger.

▪ Begin with the thumb of the left hand. First massage the top and bottom sides simultaneously and then the outer and inner sides.

▪ This is followed by massaging the index, middle, ring, and small fingers. Always start at the tip of the finger and massage down the thumb or finger, first on top and bottom, then inside and outside.

▪ Correspondingly, you will massage the toes from the tip to their basal joint later on.

■ Be sure that you always work with the pad of your thumb or index finger.

▪ Your fingernails should not dig into the tissue when massaging. With some practice, you will be able to bend your finger in an almost 90 degree angle, to use the tip of your finger to massage without pricking with short or normal nails. However, if your partner complains that you are gouging with your nails, check your massage technique. In the section entitled "Possible Reactions" (see p. 44), you will learn that sensations similar to the prick of a needle can happen even with short fingernails.

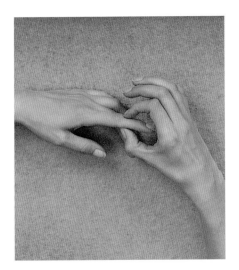

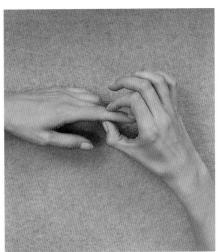

With the pinching technique, the distal joints of the thumb and index finger are straightened and the pads are pressed into the tissue without inserting the nails.

This means that if your massage technique is correct, then this sensation is just such a reaction. However, if your fingernails are slightly longer, you will have to position your thumb and index finger in a slightly more flattened fashion so as to not gouge the person massaged.

The Soothing Hold

In the course of foot reflexology, it is very well possible for the person to experience pain at some points. Each sensation of pain will tell you that the area assigned to the reflex zone is in need of some support. As long as the pain is bearable for the person concerned—be sure to ask!—continue working repeatedly with thumb or index finger on the corresponding area to deliver the healthful effects of reflexology. Doing so

means that you are massaging in a stimulating manner. If, though, the pain is very unpleasant, you can soothe the reflex zone by applying what I call the relaxation grip.

■ Ask the person to breathe deep into the belly. A useful tip here is to place the hands on the belly and to "breathe under the hands." The person massaged should tell you when the pain eases up. Relief usually follows a short time after using the relaxation grip.

■ For this, place your thumb onto the spot with the maximum sensation of pain. Go with some pressure into the tissue, pause and wait (ill. p. 34 top). For your part, concentrate on relaxed abdomen breathing as well.

■ As soon as you receive the signal that the pain has eased up, usually after about 10 to 20 seconds, slowly release the thumb. You can, if you wish, rotate on the formerly painful point with your thumb pad (ill. p. 34 bottom). Then continue with the massage.

▶
The relaxation grip is used directly on painful spots.

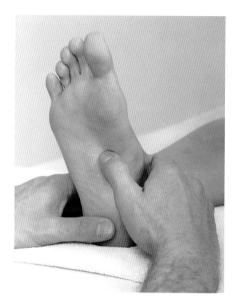

▶
The rotating motion at the end of the relaxation grip.

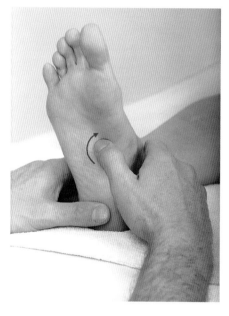

■ It rarely happens that the relaxation grip misses its effect. If it does happen, release the thumb after about 60 to 90 seconds from the reflex zone.

Stroking and Balancing Techniques

In the following, you will become familiar with different stroking movements for the foot. Stroking, like the balancing techniques, serves as a soothing alternative to the activating thumb grips.

The Energy Stroke

The energy stroke can be a good way to start your foot reflexology session, to transition from one region to the next, and even to end the treatment.

Imagine that you give your partner energy and strength with this stroking and, at the same time, that you stroke out any negative energies. The idea of giving and taking can be helpful when applying this practically, so allow the accompanying images to consciously influence your motions.

> The energy stroke is a wonderful and balancing motion. Count it, along with the thumb and index finger grips, as one of the basic tools of foot reflexology!

■ Place both palms on the bottom of the feet close to the toes. Your fingers point toward the heel, and your wrist is positioned above the foot.

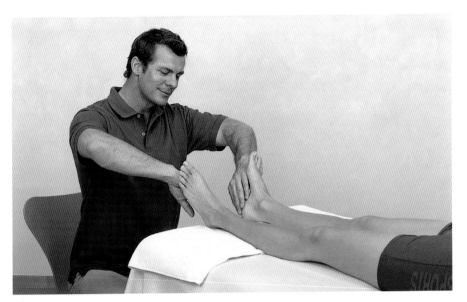

The starting
position of the
energy stroke.

- Be sure to sit straight!
- First run both hands over the sole and heel of the foot, then over the inner ankle and up the inside of the lower leg. Circle around both knees from the inside to the outside, and continue to stroke, without interruption, down on the outer lower leg and the dorsum of the foot and continue beyond the toes. Leave the big toes untouched.

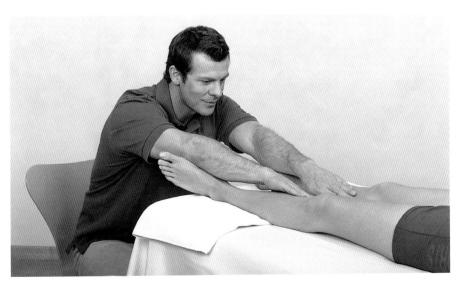

Stroke over the
inner ankles, the
lower legs, and
up to the knees.

▶

On the outer sides of the lower legs, stroke down to and over the dorsum of the feet and the toes (leave the big toes untouched).

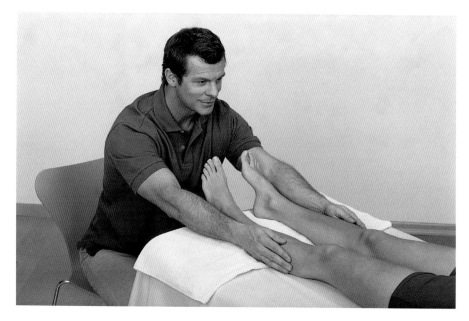

■ Your relaxed hand should cover a wider area with this stroke! Make sure that the thumb is neither standing off nor pressed onto the hand.
■ Repeat the energy stroke twice with equal pressure and with flowing movements.

▌ At first, carrying out the strokes can be confusing because the movements of each hand work in opposite directions; however, with practice, you will soon become more experienced and secure.

Make sure that you carry out these movements with an enthusiasm that comes from within.

Stretch your arms forward and your lumbar spine backward when moving upward over the legs and when going round the knees. Your pelvis should remain in contact with your chair. Feel the dynamic of your body expansion!

Do you feel that your partner finds it more pleasant if the energy stroke simply runs from the sole of the foot until just above the ankle? If so, follow through on this sensation.

Sometimes, people, particularly youngsters and men, may find the stroking of the inner side of the leg a little too intimate.

Balancing Movements

You can use balancing movements at the beginning and the end of a massage and when you switch from one region to the next.

These movements can be applied when your partner exhibits certain reactions, such as twitching and tickling (see also p. 44).

These movements serve as a balance to the activating massage work.

Stroking of the Foot

- Take the foot into both hands, one hand on top, the other at the bottom.
- Stroke over the dorsum of the foot with one hand, while simultaneously moving along the sole of the foot with the other hand.
- Work slowly! You may work synchronously with your breathing or that of your partner.
- Use the entire palm of your hand!
- You may want to repeat this simple and effective stroke several times on first one and then the other foot.

Stroking of Both Feet

- Place your palms on the dorsum of the feet while your fingers rest on the ankles.
- Now pull both hands across the dorsum of the feet toward you simultaneously.

Positioning Your Hands

- Carry out this touch with great sensitivity and awareness.
- Check your seating and posture.
- Hold the entire palm of your hand against the sole of the foot. The tips of your fingers should rest on the tips of the toes.
- Now build up the pressure slightly and consciously get in touch with the feet via your hands. All you have to do is breathe calmly and concentrate on the moment.

Left: Stroking of one foot.

Right: Stroking of both feet.

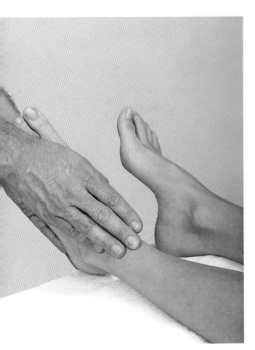

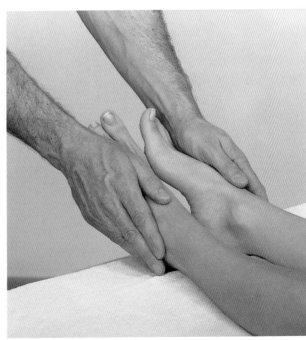

▶

Left: Placing your hands up against the feet.

Right: Holding the feet from under the heel.

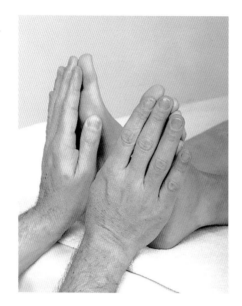

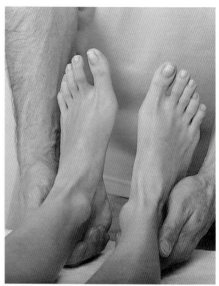

■ Relax your hands very slowly and carefully.

■ Positioning the hands against the feet is not repeated. Afterward, continue with the foot reflexology.

■ If you imagine that all the body's reflex zones are mapped out on the sole of the foot, it becomes clear that placing the palms against the feet corresponds to holding the entire human being. Therefore, this part should always be "hand"-led with special attention and great respect!

Holding the Feet from under the Heel

■ Place one hand under each foot. The heels rest in your palms, and the tips of your fingers should touch the insides of the ankles.

■ Imagine that you thus give to your partner the feeling of being able to rest, to release a burden, and to feel protected.

■ Pause for three breaths, and then continue with the massage.

If your partner places his or her trust in you, you will feel the full weight of their feet. In this instance, remember to direct your attention to your posture and to your breathing. With all the holding techniques, it is important to keep in mind the focus on your own stability. The more stable you are, the greater the foundation you will be for your partner.

Finally, holding the foot under the heel can be a very nice ending to the treatment.

Supporting One Point

After your initial massages, you might get the impression that certain points require special support. Some places on the foot feel differently than others; they may be hard, soft and fleshy, or "crunchy" like snow.

■ Zones such as these should be massaged two or three times with the stimulating thumb grip (see p. 28).

You may conclude the support as follows:

■ Hold the massaging thumb or index finger on the corresponding spot, and allow it to linger with light pressure; you may rotate slightly on the spot if you wish. Hold this for the duration of one breath.

■ Afterward, continue with the massage.

Rotating Around a Zone or Expanding the Circle

Larger areas such as the zones of the heart, liver, solar plexus, and intestine (see material beginning on pp. 61 and 67) respond well to a rotating stroke, which is a good complement to the pressure point massage. I like to use this particularly in the reflexology of the solar plexus (see p. 62).

Position the full thumb using the entire distal joint and circumscribe a spiral running in an increasing radius from the center out or work from outside to inside. Try out which direction is more suitable for you.

Consciously Carry Out Stroking and Balancing Movements

In my seminars, I constantly see participants who do not know how to continue through the course of the entire massage.

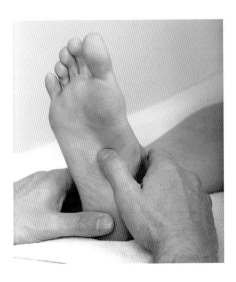

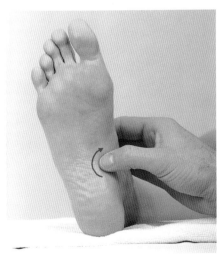

Left: Stimulating thumb grip for the support of one point.

Right: Rotation around one zone.

One stroke instinctively follows the next. A sensation that initially felt pleasant may eventually become very bothersome.

If you do not know how to continue, pause for a moment, but keep contact with the feet by holding on to them. Now calmly put your thoughts in order. Do you remember the zone chart on pages 14 and 15 and the "tilt picture" on page 12? Keep these in mind, and I assure you that you will soon remember how to continue. Another possibility is to place the zone chart next to you in the beginning (see p. 14). However, this should remain a last resort, since the temptation to constantly peek may be too great; furthermore, the "flow" that makes the massage so refreshing is lost. All there would be is a sequence of techniques instead of a holistic massage for body and soul.

▼

Stretching of the spine.

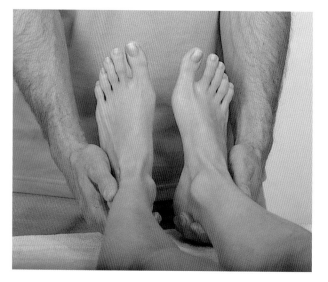

The Stretching of the Spine

The stretching described below pulls very gently on the spine. For this technique, you are not working by way of reflex zones, but rather directly on the body to effect a balance.

▪ Gently place your hands under both heels, and surround them with both hands. Do you feel the weight of the feet? Pause for a moment. The tips of your fingers now rest on the inner ankle area.

▪ Grip the heels a bit more firmly. Be certain that you are well stabilized in your seat, and concentrate on the breathing rhythm of your partner.

▪ When you sense an exhalation, increase the pressure in your palms and slowly pull the heels slightly toward you. The entire spine stretches itself.

▪ On inhalation, let go and allow the heels to settle back into their original position.

▪ You can also exert minimal pressure in the direction of the head during inhalation, but be careful that you do not push or jam!

▪ Repeat this movement with the next two breaths.

▪ If the breaths follow one another very quickly, only do the stretching with every other breath. This synchronous breathwork contributes a great deal to the support of your foot reflexology.

Massaging with the Knuckles of the Fist

The stretching of the spine is followed by a particularly powerful technique that has a balancing effect.

- Stabilize the foot with one hand by placing a supporting hand against the dorsum of the foot.
- Make a loose fist with your other hand. Use your right hand to massage the left foot, and use your left hand with the right foot.
- Position the knuckles of the fist in the groove between the toes and the ball of the foot.
- Now, with pressure, work the entire arch of the foot in semicircular movements. These movements run clockwise with the right fist and counterclockwise with the left.
- After each half-turn, position your knuckles slightly below the spot you just finished. In this way, you will work the entire arch of the foot from top to bottom, and you will end up just above the heel.

> The strength of your pressure depends on the sensitivity and age of your partner. Don't be too timid, for your massage should be felt! If you ask, you will probably find that a greater pressure is more pleasant. Think of more pressure as passing on clearer signals (i.e., greater emphasis)!

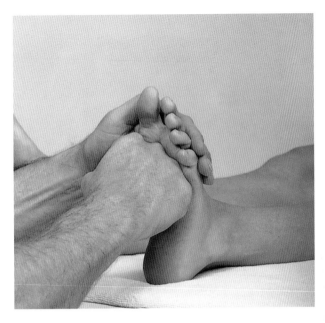

Massage with the knuckles of the fist.

Using Different Stroking and Balancing Techniques

The stroking and balancing movements introduced here can be applied randomly.

- The energy stroke, for example, is a great way to begin and end the treatment, but it also serves as a smooth transition between individual regions.
- Furthermore, the fist massage fits well into the beginning part of the treatment, after you have worked on the reflex zones of the shoulder region (see pp. 52 and 56).
- Stretching, stroking, and the laying on of hands can conclude a massage. Any of these applications are suitable when overstimulation occurs (see p. 44).

■ Alternate and experiment with what you have learned in this chapter. Be inventive!

■ However, as I have said before, do not use all the known stroke movements consecutively. That's just gilding the lily.

■ **Touching and holding—very beneficial for both sides!**

General Information Regarding Foot Reflexology

Order Therapy

Foot reflexology is counted among the forms of treatment known as order therapies, meaning that health comes from physical and psychological balance. Imbalance causes illness. A treatment that "orders" can activate a person's self-healing forces and can address an existing imbalance.

For the sake of this order, it is important that you understand the ordering principles involved.

Structure of the Foot

First of all, the massage is oriented around the anatomical structure of the foot, working with the toes and progressing forward, region after region, to the heels.

Structure of the Reflex Zones

Do you remember the theory part (see p. 10)? Zone charts and shape analogies suggest that you should massage the reflex zones of the spine, the head, and the entire torso down to the pelvis consecutively. This means that even with the sequence of the reflex zones, you should follow a fixed order, and, with the reflex zones, you are dealing with the anatomical structure of the human body.

■ **Foot reflexology regulates—both on a physical and on a psychological level.**

Therefore, do not get into the habit of picking out individual reflex zones. You cannot possibly know which part of the foot/body needs particular support. It is always good to massage the entire foot for only then does the massaged person receive the soothing feeling of "completeness."

Your Personal Order

In order to work orderly, the ordering of your own posture becomes essential. Here, I am referring to both your physical posture and your mental state. Over time and with practice, you will develop an increasingly finer feeling for both, ensuring you and your partner the greatest satisfaction.

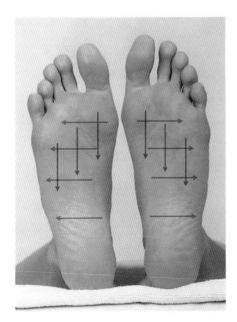

Massage Direction

The anatomy and physiology of the human body follow set directions and ordering principles. All body fluids flow in a certain direction, in the circulation of blood or the linear progression of digestion/excretion. Likewise, the direction of individual massage techniques also adhere to a clear structure. The thumb and index finger always work within a zone from top to bottom, whether in vertically or horizontally running lines. If you were to massage haphazardly, the stimulus via the reflex zones might be perceived by the person massaged as an uncomfortable muddle. When in doubt, try and ask!

■ A clear order for your procedure leads to its success!

Don't Drive in Reverse

Please take into consideration the "ordered" working direction with each massage technique. Thumb and index finger always move forward!

Intuition

With increasing practical experience, you will become steadily more aware and more sensitive to what you find on the foot. Trust your powers of observation, your sixth sense, and your intuition. The fingers will show you the right way! Rome was not built in a day, so take your time studying foot reflexology! Be patient with yourself! At the beginning, the complexity of so many aspects may confuse you: posture, massage direction, reflex zones, techniques, and stroke movements. Do you remember your first driving lesson? How complicated it seemed to think of so many things at the same time and to not make any mistakes. And now? You are an experienced and careful driver, acting almost instinctively in a correct and appropriate manner.

■ The path of learning reveals itself by practice and trial and error.

◄
The order of the foot's anatomic structure shows us the proper direction for the massage. Do not do this in "reverse"!

Breathing

Always remember to be aware of your breathing and that of your partner. Do you still feel the stress of the day? If so, your inhalation will reflect this, and you should try to establish calm breathing as this is a very important part of the treatment.

Observe your partner during the massage: if his or her breathing becomes calm and steady in the course of the treatment, this can be a sign of relaxation and well-being.

Possible Reactions

Since you activate specific stimuli in your partner, you should be aware of possible reactions during or after the treatment:
- Relaxation
- Pain in zones, signaling that an organ is not in balance
- Jerking of the feet or body
- Tickling in the feet or body
- Feeling of expansion, especially in the head
- Localized sensation of warmth in body

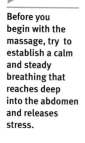

Before you begin with the massage, try to establish a calm and steady breathing that reaches deep into the abdomen and releases stress.

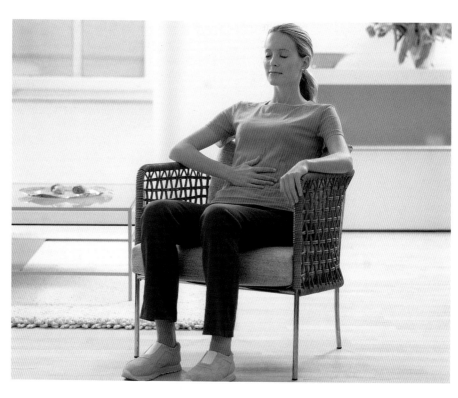

• A feeling of heaviness or lightness during and after the massage

• A relaxed well-being—this is the most common reaction after a massage

> After the massage, some people feel tired and others feel buoyant and light. Sometimes the feet are even seen differently, and the act of walking has a very different quality.

Pain

Sensations of pain can be of various kinds: pricking, dull, or stabbing, depending on the points massaged.

Use such reactions as the occasion to focus your efforts on the affected area on the foot. What reflex zone are you dealing with?

In general, each reaction of pain is a suggestion that something is out of balance in the corresponding reflex zone. For you, this means that you should pay careful attention to the corresponding area by massaging the affected area one or two more times.

Sweating

If the massaged person begins to sweat, gets moist hands or feet, or even a suddenly dry mouth, then the body is signaling that the current stimuli are too much and that it needs a rest. React by applying one of the light, relaxing stroking techniques (see p. 34).

If you exhibit these symptoms yourself, you should do the same. You most likely have worn yourself out! Allow yourself some rest during the massage by tackling the whole affair with a greater sense of peace. A few stroking techniques and less pressure—and your tension will soon drop to normal.

The "Where It" Rule with Pain

You will work where it hurts. My teacher Renate Roelofs from Cologne calls this the "Where It" rule. Makes sense, doesn't it?

This simple rule basically means that you give special care and attention to painful points of the corresponding zone. Pain is always a signal to "take care of it." You should by all means observe this.

Do All Zones Feel Equally?

With time, you will notice that the foot can be a very complex area (see p. 39). There are warm or cool feet and sometimes only a part of the foot is warm while another is cold. Become familiar with all these characteristics of the feet!

Ticklish Feet?

Your friend tells you with a tone that runs from warning to threatening: "I am very ticklish on the feet!" Take careful note of this. Avoid the stroking touches at the beginning, and be sure that the foot is well supported. The pressure of thumb or index finger should be clear and determined.

It is important that you proceed from the assumption that your foot reflexology does not tickle. If, however, the treatment tickles beyond the initial stage, you will have to stop. Generally speaking, though, any tickling sensation tends to subside rather quickly.

Need to End the Massage Abruptly?

What if you have to end the massage early? In this case, with both hands, reach around the outer side of both feet from the right and the left; applying a short pressure signals farewell, much like a handshake (see p. 74), and your massage is finished.

Insistent or Gentle Pressure?

The pressure point massage is given with continuous pressure. At the beginning, we tend to work in a rather reserved manner. The contact is subsequently blurred, and clear information is missing. Be sure to ask if you are not sure if your grip is too firm or too loose. Stroke movements, if applicable, are carried out gently.

■ With the massage, you should not press too firmly nor grip too loosely. Our "grip" signals the quality of our massage presence.

▶

If you need to end the massage early, give a farewell with a short pressure of the hand—best if following a stroking movement.

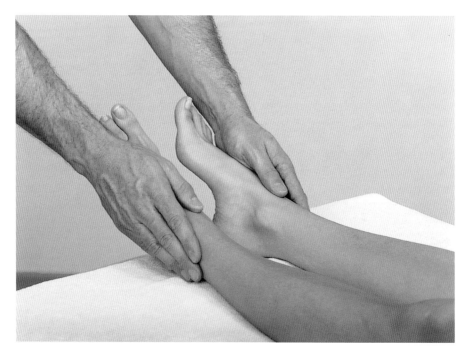

Fast or Slow?

Despite all the tranquility, we are always active during foot reflexology. This activity should be felt in the work speed. However, be attentive to yourself, and slow down when you notice that you start to rush. Each massage point must be treated individually!

Cover the Feet?

Carefully covering the foot that is not currently being worked on always feels pleasant and thoughtful. You should first cover the foot just massaged, then uncover the other. The first foot is now allowed to rest and may withdraw under the blanket.

Massaging the Feet Simultaneously or Consecutively?

The feet can be treated either simultaneously or consecutively.

Simultaneous Massage of the Feet

The reflex zones of the spine, thyroid gland, heart, kidneys, pancreas, solar plexus, and the small intestine can be easily massaged simultaneously via both feet just like the zone of the pelvic floor. These zones are located on the sole of the foot, and the organs are positioned in pairs (kidneys), placed in the middle of the body (spine, thyroid gland, heart), or stretched across the left or right side of the body (pancreas, solar plexus, intestine, pelvic floor).

Because of the steady and synchronized alternating of work and resting phases, it's easy to get into the swing of a rhythmic, dynamic massage when working simultaneously with both thumbs.

After a few massages, you will establish a good, straight posture, with feet firmly rooted on the ground, and nice, easy, yet thorough technique.

Massaging First One Then the Other Foot

With ailments such as a cold or flu, it works better to massage the reflex zones for each foot individually. In this way, you devote significant time to the respective zones.

The same applies for the zone of the solar plexus, which is best addressed by treating first the reflex area of one foot and then immediately moving to the same reflex area of the second foot, thus treating the particular reflex zone consecutively.

When to Change Feet?

Beginning on page 10, I introduced Fitzgerald's zones. Switch the foot being massaged after having worked one of Fitzgerald's levels, if you are not massaging both feet simultaneously. Starting with the reflex zone of the spine on the inner edge of the foot and the massaging of the toes, you will then massage each region consecutively, moving back and forth between the feet. This is presented in fuller detail starting on page 49.

While performing a simultaneous massage, the shift to consecutive treatment always happens at the particular points of massage when a singular treatment is advisable. Anything dealing with the reflex zones of the toes, the dorsum, and the outer ankles are counted among these singular treatments. The reason is purely technical: Neither toes nor the dorsum of the foot can be sufficiently stabilized during a simultaneous massage. Likewise the reflex zones of the colon have to be massaged consecutively first on the right, then on the left foot since digested food travels exactly like this through the intestine.

When Does the Right and When Does the Left Thumb Massage?

Both thumbs are used alternately. If you find that the massage becomes unwieldy, simply switch hands to obtain a more comfortable working position.

Get used to massaging with first one thumb and then the other, keeping in mind that it is always important that you can reach the appropriate zone in a straight and comfortable posture. A good "rule of thumb" is to use the right hand for the left foot and the left hand on the right foot.

It also works out well if you treat the inner half of the foot with the one thumb and the outer half with the other.

Supporting the Foot

The supporting hand is always close to the working thumb. The consistent touch of both hands is a reassuring contact, which strengthens the trust implicit in the massage through these clear and reassuring signals. Of course, this means support in both a literal and a figurative sense.

Observe the Following Principles

- Check your posture repeatedly.
- Be attentive to your partner's needs and reactions.
- Control the rhythm and intensity of your hands, thumbs, and fingers.
- Allow sufficient time to become familiar with the many different reflex zones.
- The worth of a massage is determined not only by the number of reflex points massaged, but also by the concentration, the calm, and the devotion, shaped by rhythm and dynamic, that you bring to the experience.

Foot Reflexology—
Zones and Organs

Before you begin with the foot reflexology, consider for a moment about how long the treatment should last. In this way, you can plan to do justice to all the areas on the feet.

Beginning the Massage— The Greeting

The first thing to do is to establish contact.
▪ Place your hands lightly on the lower legs or feet of your partner.
▪ Direct your attention to yourself, to your posture, and to your breathing before attending to your partner.
▪ Pause for a moment to establish contact, since the person receiving the massage likewise needs to become accustomed to the situation.
▪ The energy stroke is a perfect introduction to the massage (see p. 34).

Do you have the impression that your partner cannot unwind easily? Suggest that he close his eyes. Keep in mind, though, that some people are uneasy if they cannot see what is going on around them.

Region 1

The Inner Edge of the Foot

The massage of the inner edges of both feet follows after two or three energy strokes.
▪ Position your thumbs from top right and left on the inside of the big toes. The fingers rest level with the toe line on the dorsum of the foot, the fingertips point outward, and your elbows are drawn slightly in.

▼
Top:
The thumb works, while the other fingers rest loosely on top.

Bottom:
This is the correct posture of the hands. You will see the precise order of reflex points on the following pages.

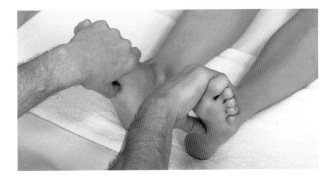

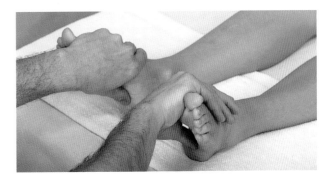

- While your fingers stabilize the foot from above, the thumbs work along the inner edges of the feet. You can get your bearings by the clearly tangible metatarsal bones on both sides as you work your way downward.
- Don't massage the bones, but rather the spaces next to them!
- The zone treatment stops at the lower edge of the heel where no bone can be felt.
- Repeat this part of the massage one or two more times.
- If it seems too complicated to massage both feet at once, address them one at a time. Hold the foot with your free hand from the outer side and support it well. Be sure that you always work in the same direction from the toes to the heels: from top to bottom.

Uncontrolled changes of direction can lead to unconscious irritations in your partner.

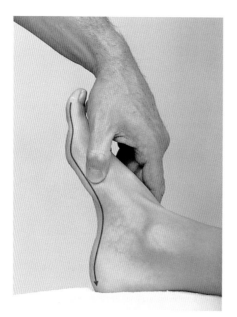

The thumb massages below the bone edges along the inner foot.

- Most likely, you will have to pull your chair slightly to the side in order to sit comfortably in front of the respective foot. Remember to cover the other foot carefully.
- You may conclude your massage with a discretionary one to three energy strokes.

Zones That Are Influenced by This Massage

The massage from the big toe via the basal joints of the toe, the ball, and the inner arch down to the heel works consecutively on the reflex zones of the neck, breast, spinal column, and sacrum. In this way, the entire back is massaged all the way through, and you are devoting a great deal of necessary attention to the spinal column.

Painful Points

In case painful spots appear in the area treated, repeat the massage at that point, keeping in mind the intensity of the pressure: neither too timid nor too vigorous. Remember that pain indicates the body's need for special attention within the framework of foot reflexology (the "Where It" rule).

If the pain becomes unpleasant, change your strategy and adjust to a soothing hold (see p. 33).

The Toes and the Upper Transverse Arch

Next, the toes are massaged, including the pads, the space between the toes, and the upper transverse arch.
- Cover the left foot with a blanket or a towel while treating the right foot with soothing stroking movements.
- The massaging hand keeps the upper part of the foot well supported.

Turning and Stretching the Toes

This is an exercise to loosen and relax the toes.
- Start with the big toe. Support the upper foot with one hand, and, using the thumb and index finger of the other hand, surround the toe at the bottom, just above the basal joint.
- Now, rotate the toe slowly. Notice how it feels when you make larger circles that seek to encompass the room. Then, gradually reduce the radius to very, very small circles, which would not even be noticed by an onlooker and are only felt by you and your partner.
- The toe on the left foot should be turned clockwise, the right foot counterclockwise.
- Continue by repeating the rotation on the next toe. It is easy to transition from toe to toe fluidly. Simply allow the movements to run from outside to inside, and from greater to smaller circles. Do not jump back and forth since this can instill a feeling of unrest.
- After you have addressed all the toes from the first foot in this way, you can stretch each toe. Grab the basal joint deeply, and stretch one toe after the other with only a slight amount of force. It is important that you hold each of the toes the entire time by the joint and stabilize them.

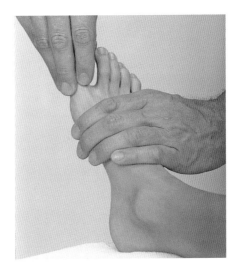

Rotating the toes: Stabilize the foot with the supporting hand. Reach around the toes to grip the basal joints.

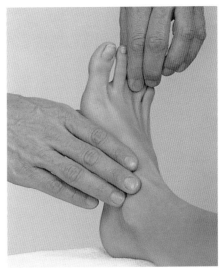

Stretching the toes: Here, you also grab the toes by the basal joints.

▶

Left:
Massaging of the pads of the toes.

Right:
Stroking the area between the toes by holding the web of skin.

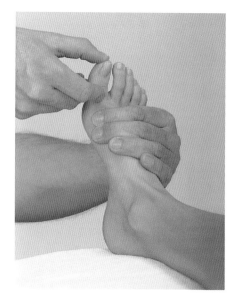

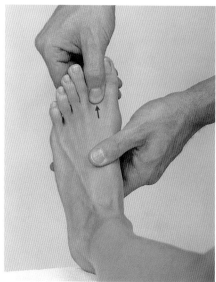

If the foot reflexology treatment is supposed to be brief, then you may forgo rotating and stretching the toes.

Massaging the Toes

For this, you can work either with the thumb and index finger or you may use the pinching technique (see p. 32). See which suits you best.

■ Each toe is massaged from top and bottom, from the inside and the outside, but you can omit the toenails. Always repeat the same order with each toe.

■ Then massage the pads of the toes with the thumb grip—usually two grips on each toe.

■ It is possible to treat the big toe (in the sense of "one for all") as the representative of all toes. If initial massages demonstrate that you need a lot of time for the toes, you should practice this occasionally. The same applies for giving a brief massage (see p. 83).

Massaging the Spaces between the Toes

There are small webs of skin between the toes that are massaged after the pads.

■ Take each little web between your thumb and index finger and stroke it. Begin with the big toe, and end with the small toe.

Transverse Arch

After you are done massaging the toes, dedicate some time to the area below the toes, the upper transverse arch.

■ Here, you can either massage with one hand moving from the outside edge to the inside edge, or you may choose to work with both hands. When working with both hands, both thumbs move inward toward one another.

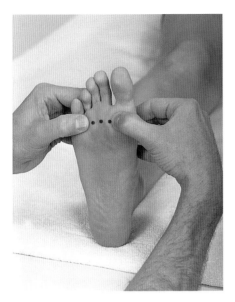

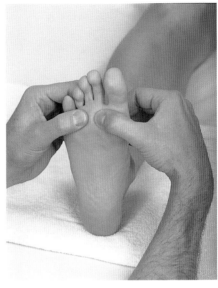

Left:
Massage below the toes.

Right:
Both thumbs move toward one another.

Massage with the Rubbing Technique

■ Start on the outer side of the knuckle joint of the small toe.
■ With the outer edge of a slightly flexed index finger, rub along the outer edge of the foot. Exert pressure!
■ Work downward about a third of the length of the foot.
■ Repeat the rubbing technique two or three times, keeping the index finger flexed.

Massage with the Knuckles of the Fist

The description for the practical execution of this method is found on page 41 under "Using Different Stroking and Balancing Techniques."
■ The movement of pressure and turning often has a "cheering" effect. However, while the position of your knuckles and the turn of the fist in the arch of the foot should be enthusiastic in adults, with children under six years of age you should be more careful.

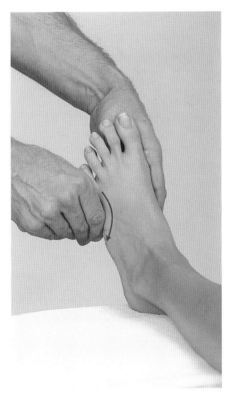

The rubbing technique is achieved through the pressure exerted by the outer edge of the index finger.

Massaging the Second Foot

■ After massaging the first foot, cover it carefully. Then uncover the second foot.

■ Remember: Any jerky, impetuous movements can upset your carefully planned dynamic-rhythmic massage.

■ The massage of the second foot may be quite similar to that of the first; of course, it may also be a complete surprise. It can very well happen that different areas on the left and the right feet are sensitive to pain. If you find such a reaction, repeat your treatment of the spot in question (the "Where It" rule).

■ Finally, giving an energy stroke to both feet at the same time can be a great way to wrap up (see p. 34).

Zones Influencing This Massage

Use the tilt picture (see p. 12) and zone chart (see pp. 14 and 15) to help you. Observe the sitting profile, and you will recognize how the back runs. If you apply Fitzgerald's zones, you see that the spine is found in zone 1 on the foot. The foot profile also suggests that the area of the head is mapped both in the big toe and in the other toes. Thus the big toe acts as the reflex zone for all areas of the head and can be massaged as a representative for all toes.

When you encircle the toes, a feeling of relaxation arises either generally through the body or more specifically in the head. Think of the stretching as making space in the overcrowded head. Nonetheless, you should be careful with people who have a tendency to get headaches or migraines when you work on reflex zones assigned to the head. Any pressure should be increased slowly; this gradual intensity often leads to a relief in the symptoms.

Pituitary Gland

The reflex zone of the pituitary gland is located in the middle of the crown of the big toe. This part of the brain controls the hormonal system. Growth, energy regulation, stress processing, immune system, procreation—all these are coordinated through hormones, which, balanced with one another, react very sensitively to disturbances. With a massage of this reflex zone, you can support the work of the pituitary gland.

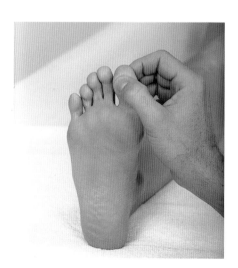

The reflex zone of the pituitary gland is positioned on what we call the crown of the big toe.

Teeth

The zones above and below the interphalangeal joints of the toes correspond to the teeth. The upper jaw reflex zone lies above, and the lower jaw below the joints. For those people who tend to grind their teeth both literally and figuratively, reflexology is certainly beneficial. With periodontitis, for example, the massage supports the sensitive jaw region.

Palatal Tonsils

If the person suffers from a sore throat, the reflex zone of the palatal tonsil on the lower inner side of the big toe will often be sensitive to pain. Therefore, you can either massage it with the thumb grip or, if the pain is stronger, you can address it with the soothing hold (see p. 33).

Eyes

You can also massage the reflex zones of the eyes on the second and third toes. Treat the appropriate toe from both the top and the bottom. If your partner tends to keep his or her "eyes closed" to ideas (i.e., be close-minded), the massage of the eye reflex zone can be helpful. In addition, if there is an eyesight defect, you support the existing vision.

Ears

The zone of the ear is actually outside the body. Look at the tilt picture (see p. 12), and determine the approximate location of the ear reflex zone

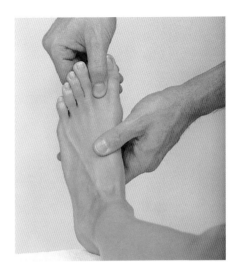

◄

The zone of the palatal tonsils on the inner edge of the big toe can react with pain as part of the lymphatic system.

before you go on reading. On the zone chart, if you trace the corresponding longitudinal zone down to the toe, you will arrive at the space between the second-to-last and the last toes. Here, you will find the reflex zones for the inner, middle, and outer ears. The inner and middle ears' reflex zone is on the second-to-last toe on the lateral outer side, while the outer ear is on the small toe, all the way down on the inner edge.

A sensitive ear reflex zone can indicate an oncoming inflammation of the middle ear. This can often be observed when massaging young children. The antibodies that are naturally produced in the body are stimulated through reflexology. Once again, if there is a strong reaction to pain, you should use the soothing hold (see p. 33).

Upper Lymphatic System

With the stroking of the small webs of skin between the toes, you will stimulate the lymphatic system of the head and neck regions, which will in turn strengthen the body's immune system. The swollen lymph nodes that signal an oncoming cold will be reflected in sensitivity between the toes. This sensitivity can also appear with allergy sufferers. The work on these zones needs only a slight pressure to be effective.

Nasal Sinuses

The nasal sinuses have their reflex zone on top of the pads of the toes. This is effective against the symptoms of colds, stuffy nose, and sinusitis.

Cervical Spine

The cervical spine as a reflex zone runs along the basal joint of the big toe. It is often massaged at the beginning of the session. You may choose to pay particular attention to this zone when your partner is experiencing tension in the neck and shoulder area.

Thyroid Gland

The thyroid gland is located in the neck, and the assigned reflex zone is found in the lower neck of the big toe. Massage the zone at the juncture between the big toe and the ball of the foot. The hormones produced in the thyroid gland are important for mental and physical development. A massage here can have a relaxing effect when your partner is active and a stimulating effect when he or she is lethargic.

The parathyroid glands neighboring the thyroid affect the phosphate and calcium levels of the blood by means of the parathyroid hormone produced there. Reflexology can stimulate bone formation through stimulation of this point.

Shoulders

When you look at the form analogy, you will recognize the shoulder area on the foot. Our shoulders frequently carry a great deal of tension owing to the worries and stresses caused by our single-minded work at the office or in school. Treat the reflex zone with the awareness that you are also massaging the shoulders and the neck!

Shoulder Joint and Upper Arm

The palpable, visible metacarpophalangeal joint of the little toe is the starting point for the rubbing technique on the foot's outer edge. As a reflex zone, this joint corresponds to the shoulder joint, while the outer edge of the foot corresponds to the upper arm. If there is pain in the shoulder

▶

Massage reflex points in region 1:
1a Cervical spine
1b Thoracic spine
1c Lumbar spine
1d Sacrum
1e Tailbone
 2 Pituitary
   gland
 3 Thyroid gland
 4 Palatal tonsils
 5 Eyes
 6 Ears
 7 Teeth
 8 Sinuses
 9 Lymph in the
   head area
10 Shoulder
   region

joint, you can try to alleviate it through foot reflexology. The treatment of this reflex zone is often reported as being a particularly pleasant experience (see "rubbing technique," p. 53). I'm certain that you are familiar with the kind of pain that does not actually hurt but that is still unpleasant and difficult to pinpoint. The rubbing technique works particularly well on just such pain.

Summary of Region 1 Massage

Based on the organs described and their respective zones, it is obvious how dense the connections are in the head area. The bony structures of the skull and jaw, the teeth, the sense organs such as eyes and ears, the hormonal system including the pituitary and thyroid glands, and the lymphatic throat ring, are all very closely positioned. Therefore, you should be cautious when it comes to making a categorical or linear assignment of body-reflex zones, since these, too, are placed closely together. A great deal of knowledge and experience is needed for a diagnostic use of reflexology. Rather, you should limit yourself to the "Where It" rule, so that when you work with concentration and inner rest, you will find a lot of joy in simply massaging without trying to diagnose pain, organs, or illness.

> Your job is to give relaxation, well-being, and a strengthening of body and soul. Any concern about "What point was that?" should be of secondary importance only.

Region 2

The Dorsum of the Foot

Now we continue with the practical work on the dorsum, or the top, of the foot. Generally, the feet are massaged one after the other, since there would not be enough support if worked on simultaneously.

Massaging the dorsum of the foot is actually quite simple since the metatarsal bones show you the way.

■ Start on the right side, and leave the left foot covered.

■ Begin with the area between the big and second toes and work along between the bones by using the thumb grip, up to approximately the middle of the dorsum of the foot. The end of your "path" is where the midtarsal joints of the foot begin.

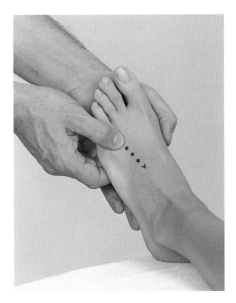

◄ Reflexology on the dorsum of the foot: Massage from inside to outside along the space between the metatarsal bones.

■ Using this pattern, successively massage all four "grooves" between the metatarsal bones.
■ However, before you move on to the next groove, repeat the massage once or twice.
■ Be sure to massage the spaces between and not on the bones.
■ When working on the dorsum of the foot, you will probably have to shift your seat to better reach the outside of the foot. Instead of reaching around, you should always sit upright and relaxed and in direct line with the foot.

Ventilating

What I like to call "ventilating" is well suited for bringing the treatment of the dorsum of the foot to a close.
■ Take each foot by its midpoint into your hands. The tips of your fingers rest on the dorsum of the foot between the metatarsal bones of the first and second toes. The balls of the hands support the foot from below.

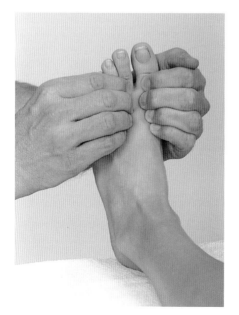

▶
The metatarsal bones are displaced against each other when "ventilating."

■ By alternating the right and left hand in pressing away from your body, the metatarsal bones are moved both against and away from each other. Your movement is precipitated by the heels of the hands, and the tips of your fingers continuously adjust to and support the displacing rhythm.
■ After you have displaced ("ventilated") the first and second metatarsal bones three times, move outward to the next space, then to the third, and finally to the fourth space in between.
■ Finally, take the foot between both hands and stroke it with enthusiasm.
■ Afterward, change to the other foot.

Zones That Are Influenced by This Massage

When you look at the zone chart of Dr. Fitzgerald (see pp. 14 and 15) or the analogy of the body depicted in the perpendicular foot (see p. 12), you will find the reflex zones of the dorsum of the foot as images of the ribs and the rib cage. This becomes easy to remember if you imagine the vertically running metatarsal bones as corresponding to the horizontally running ribs.

Lungs and Bronchia

Via the foot reflexology of the dorsum of the foot, you will address the lungs and bronchia.

Although the various reflex zones of the rib cage can be massaged both from the top (on the dorsum) and from the bottom (on the sole), practical experience has shown that it is useful to concentrate on massaging the dorsum when treating the bronchia.

The lobes of the lungs and the fine branches of the bronchia are organs that are responsible for the body's oxygen supply: "I can't catch my breath," "everything feels closed," and "I can't breathe" are familiar expressions of stress and tension, thus making clear to us the significance of "drawing breath" as a giver of life and energy.

With firmness and rhythm, massage the dorsum of the foot. People with allergies often react sensitively in this reflex zone. For problems such as asthma, recurrent cough, or general weakness, these reflex zones are a good starting point for support and strength.

With acute troubles, work with very slight pressure or even limit yourself to merely holding the dorsum. For this, hold the foot both top to bottom using both hands. Pause for two or three exhalations. Exert slight pressure onto the sole and dorsum with your palms, and then loosen your hands. Holding the reflex zone area of the lungs and bronchia is often very pleasurable.

"Ventilating" corresponds to the airing of individual sections of the lungs. Imagine this: Just as you may air out a blanket, so fresh wind streams into your lungs. Through displacing, you bring movement to areas of the lungs that normally are not frequently moved or aired out—and movement and "fresh air" never hurt!

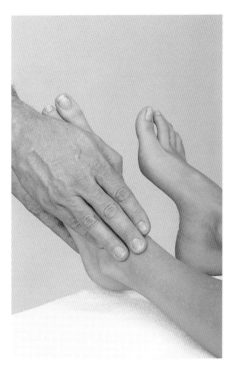

◀
The holding and stroking of the dorsum touches the reflex zones of lungs and bronchia.

When stroking the dorsum of the foot with one hand from the top or with both hands from top and bottom, envision the pleasant feeling of someone comfortably rubbing the back and ribs of a person suffering from a cough and the sniffles.

Region 3

The Sole of the Foot

After massaging the dorsum, turn to the sole of the foot. The treatment of the following zones can be carried out either on each foot consecutively or on both feet simultaneously. In the latter case, the right thumb massages the left foot and the left thumb the right one. Your palms rest on the inner edges of the foot, and the fingers are loosely positioned on the dorsum.

With some practice, synchronously massaging both feet like this will become easy. The advantage with concentrating on the sole is that the pressure applied by the thumbs can be felt throughout the entire body as a vibration or oscillation. This vibration continues up the big, long bones of the legs, through the spine, and up to the head. Observe how the head slightly moves along in the rhythm of the massage.

If you are a beginner, though, it is best to tackle the feet one at a time. In this way, you practice and concentrate first on one and then on the other foot.

■ The left foot remains covered while you carefully uncover the right one.

■ Using the thumb grip, massage your way from the ball of the foot to just below the big toe in vertical or horizontal lines. When doing so, always begin on the inner edge.

■ If there is pain, use less pressure or change to the soothing hold (p. 33).

■ Make certain that you always massage from the heel toward the toes and from the inside to the outside.

■ Use either the right or the left thumb as you see fit, and determine for yourself where which hand works better.

■ In the area of the ball, a rotating pressure (p. 39) can be used. Position the thumb, exert pressure on the spot, and then move the tissue under the pad of your thumb in a circular movement: rotate counterclockwise on the right foot and clockwise on the left foot.

Left:
The simultaneous massage of both feet.

Right:
The one-sided massage of the ball region on the right foot.

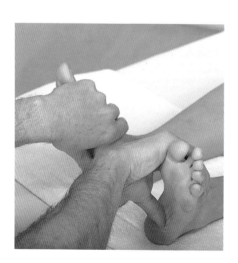

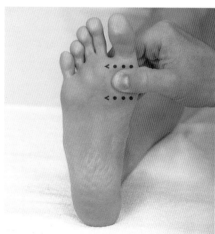

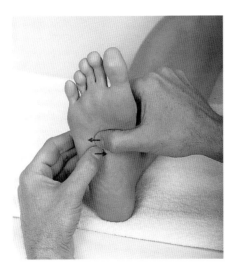

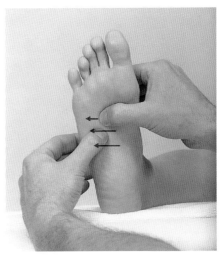

Left:
There are two possibilities in massaging the reflex zone of the liver (see p. 63): On the right sole of the foot, both thumbs massage toward one another or...

Right:
The left hand supports and the right thumb massages—from inside to outside, from bottom to top.

■ Repeat the massage of the ball once or twice.
■ Next work the entire upper arch of the foot. Use the illustrations to determine which zones are treated. Massage the outer part of the right foot first (ill. above).

■ Then change to the inner edge and massage below the ball at a distance of approximately two fingers in and down (ill. bottom left).
■ The next zone is located approximately a thumb's width below; it runs horizontally in the sole of the foot (ill. bottom right).

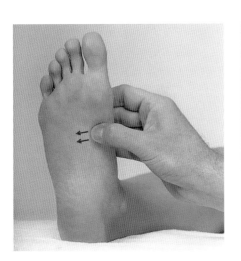

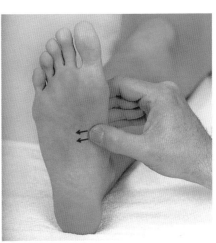

Left:
Reflex zone of the stomach (see p. 64).

Right:
Reflex zone of the pancreas (see p. 65).

▷

Left:
Radial massage on both feet simultaneously.

Right:
Radial massage first on the right and then on the left foot (see p. 65, solar plexus).

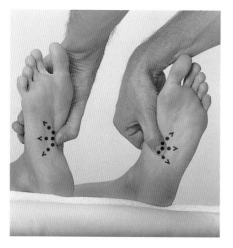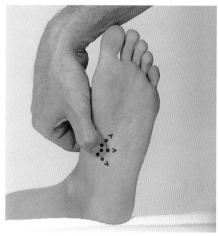

▽ ▷

Left:
Massage of the kidney reflex zone.

Middle:
Massage of the urethra reflex zone.

Right:
Massage of the bladder reflex zone.

■ Now comes a radial massage pattern. Below the previous zone and overlapping it slightly, massage the sole of the foot along three radial paths (ill. above).

■ Repeat the radial path twice more.

■ Next position your thumb in between the third and fourth metatarsal bones at a distance of two fingers width below the ball. Then, consecutively carry out the thumb grip in a radius of approximately three-quarters of an inch (two centimeters) as you eventually wander in a crescent moon toward the heel (ill. bottom from left to right).

■ This massage path concludes with a couple of pressure grips just above the beginning of the heel on the inner edge of the foot.

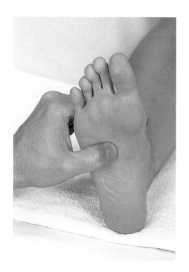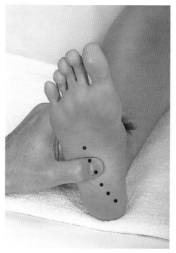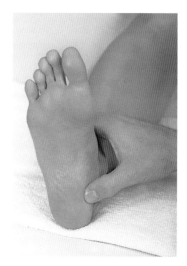

Zones That Are Influenced by This Massage

Again, look at the connections indicated by Dr. Fitzgerald's zones, or you can recognize them in the form analogy. The thyroid, heart, and lungs are positioned more or less concentrically; this is followed by the liver, with the gallbladder in the upper right abdomen, the spleen at the left. In the center lie the stomach, pancreas, and the branched solar plexus. Laterally, right and left, you will find the kidneys and the urethra running down to the bladder.

Thyroid Gland

The reflex zone of the thyroid gland lies on the path from the big toe to the ball of the foot. We have already elaborated on its significance in the explanation of the head reflex zones (see p. 56).

You support the thyroid gland's work by massaging the reflex zone two to three times with the thumb grip from top to bottom and from inside to outside.

Similarly, the thyroid is also affected by a general massage of the big toe.

Heart

The reflex zones of the heart are located on the ball of the foot. Due to the slightly left-leaning tilt to the heart, you can massage a bit more to the outside on the left foot.

The center of the body's circulation, the muscles of the heart tirelessly pump blood through the body, providing oxygen and nutrients to the largest organs and to the smallest cells. Emotionally, the

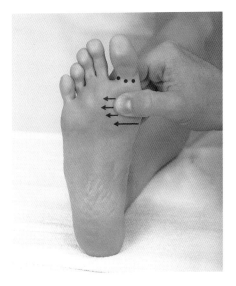

Massaging the reflex zones of thyroid and heart on the right foot.

heart is also the seat of our feelings. Think of sayings such as "a broken heart," "heartfelt greetings," "with all my heart," and "pouring your heart out" to someone you trust. Clearly, the heart is much more than just a well-toned hollow muscle!

So take all this into consideration when the respective reflex zone reacts sensitively to the massage.

Particularly with heartache, a calming touch of your palm against the heart zone and a gentle pressure massage feel reassuring. Once again, pay close attention to your own breathing.

Liver, Gall Ducts, Gallbladder

Because of the position of these organs in the abdomen region, massaging the right foot may differ from the left in the areas between the ball of the foot and the heel.

In the right upper abdomen below the costal arch, the liver stretches across the entire width. Although a corner juts into the left upper abdomen, we will pass over this part since the stomach region is positioned in the same place. Toward the bottom of the liver, you will find the gallbladder. With foot reflexology, both the gall ducts and the gallbladder are treated within the framework of the liver zone.

Look at the zone chart, and use the perpendicular foot to orient yourself when locating the liver and gall zone.

The liver is a significant detoxification organ, and, together with the gallbladder, it is part of the digestive system. They play a significant role in our well-being. Stimulating this reflex zone supports the functions of the liver and gallbladder. Problems of indigestion or troubles due to gallstones can be addressed through foot reflexology. Emotionally, we understand that feelings such as envy, defiance, and jealousy are assigned to these organs; therefore, a massage of the feet in this reflex zone can have a detoxifying effect on us both physically and mentally.

Spleen

The spleen is located in the left abdominal area behind the stomach and above and behind the left kidney. Much smaller than the liver, the spleen is an important organ of lymphatic defense and protects the body from germs by antibodies, so a pressure point massage in this area can strengthen the body's immune system.

For people suffering from allergies or weak constitutions, the spleen's reflex zone should always be included in the treatment. The same holds true for massaging the reflex zones of the upper lymph system (see p. 56) and the lymph ducts of the pelvic region (see p. 72).

Stomach

Following the esophagus, the stomach lies in the upper abdomen between the liver and the spleen and just above the pancreas. Since the stomach is slightly stretched toward the right side, massage of the reflex zone of the stomach is treatable on both feet, however, the right foot has a more expansive area.

Children easily get a "belly ache" when they get overexcited. But adults also often react with stomach pain when stressed or worried, with an acidic stomach or even a painful ulcer as a result. The irritated stomach wall, excess stomach acid, and even heartburn require loving care via our feet. A massage of the stomach reflex zone can bring relief and simultaneously produce a feeling of calm.

Foot reflexology is not about picking and choosing a few specific zones. The full benefit of the massage unfolds through treating the entire person, both physically and mentally, via the entire foot!

Pancreas

The pancreas is located slightly below and behind the stomach and thus responds well to the reflexology of other organs in the same area. Since the pancreas stretches across the abdomen, from right to left, the reflex zones of the pancreas are massaged on both the left and right foot.

The pancreas has two tasks: First, it secretes digestive enzymes into the small intestine, aiding the digestion of food. Second, the vital hormone insulin is produced here. This is absolutely necessary for processing absorbed carbohydrates. Problems with insulin levels can lead to diabetes.

For persons with diabetes, you should spend extra time on the pancreas zone. Of course, an existing condition of diabetes cannot be cured through reflexology. However, caring for the feet can provide a measure of stability for the person. This feeling cannot be undervalued when it comes to chronic diseases.

Encourage digestion with a rhythmical-dynamic massage.

Solar Plexus

Now we are coming to the solar plexus, which you have already worked radially during your massage. The solar plexus is widely branched and supplies the inner organs with nerve impulses, so it plays a central role in many meditative exercises and techniques. Massaging this reflex zone affects the entire nervous system. A stimulating or soothing hold can have an invigorating or relaxing effect.

You will find the starting point for this massage on the inner edge of the foot. As you move your thumb along the edge, you will discover a small "hollow" in the middle of the foot: a gap between the metatarsal and cuneiform bones. Starting from this point, massage in a radial pattern into the foot.

For tension or nervousness—even restlessness in children—work soothingly and hold your thumbs or the palms of your hands against the solar plexus reflex zone. Massage with gentle pressure only. If you are addressing a lack of drive, tiredness, or dullness, you can work a bit more firmly and in a more rhythmic and dynamic fashion. Trust your intuition—it will guide you in the right direction!

Massaging and "holding" the area of the solar plexus can have noticeable effects in the body. People often mention feelings of warmth and tickling or a pleasant sensation of flowing energy. The involuntary nervous system also reacts to the treatment. Holding and massaging might even have a stabilizing effect on you! However, remember to continue to pay close attention to your own posture and relaxed breathing!

Kidneys, Urethra, Urinary Bladder

The kidneys are positioned right and left of the spine, and above the hips. Through their production of urine, they represent an important excretory organ. The enzyme renin, created in the kidneys, affects the electrolyte level and blood pressure.

With kidney problems and bladder infections, you should only work with gentle pressure and balancing movements (see p. 34). With fever, you might want to avoid pressure points entirely in the course of foot reflexology. You can always perform holding techniques and stroking movements. For people who have a tendency to bladder infections, as well as children who are wetting their beds, perform a stimulating massage in the intervals free of symptoms; in this way, you can work on the kidney zones, including the reflex line of the urethra.

Conclude your attention to the kidneys with a massage of the urinary bladder zone. It is positioned on the inner edge of the foot approximately at the beginning of the heel. When under stress, it often appears as a small pad. The kidney reflex zone and the zones of the urethra and bladder can easily be massaged synchronously on both feet.

Summary of the Massage for Region 3

The reflex zones of region 3 correspond to the area of the upper abdomen, upward through the heart region and downward through the urethra and bladder. Here you will encounter many organs: liver, gallbladder, spleen, stomach, pancreas, and solar plexus. Do not get frustrated if you do not detect all the zones with the initial massages. I assure you that with each new treatment you will become more and more secure in the techniques and more experienced in the knowledge of individual zones.

▶
Massage reflex zones in region 3:
 3 Thyroid gland
13 Heart
14 Liver/gall-
    bladder
15 Spleen
16 Stomach
17 Pancreas
18 Solar plexus
19 Kidneys
20 Urethra
21 Urinary
    bladder

Region 4

The Bottom Part of the Sole

Now follows the massage of another part of
the foot sole. The fourth region is bounded
by the end of the metatarsal—and the beginning
of the tarsal bones—and the beginning of the
heel. You are familiar already with the upper
part where the solar plexus is located (see
region 3, p. 65).

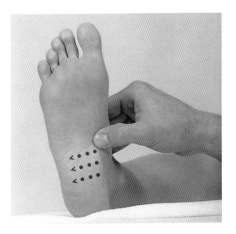

Massaging one
foot with one
thumb.

Massage of One Foot

- Work with both thumbs simultaneously by
moving toward one another from the right and
from the left.
- If you prefer to massage this area of the sole
with only one thumb, then you should use the
other hand to support the foot and work from
inside to outside and from top to bottom.

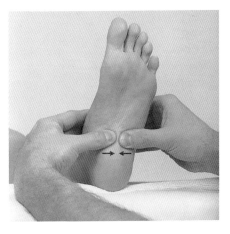

Massaging
one foot with
both thumbs
simultaneously.

Massaging Both
Feet Simultaneously

- Beginning on the inner edge of the feet,
massage with both thumbs right and left simultaneously.
- Work in perpendicular lines and in a calm
rhythm until you reach the outer edge. Your
fingers should rest loosely on the dorsum of
the foot.

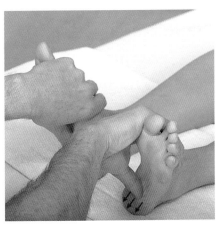

Massaging
both feet
simultaneously.

> This simultaneous treatment of the center
> points of the soles conveys the massage
> rhythm to the entire body.

▷
Massaging the right foot—outer edge and upper margin of region 4. The left thumb massages.

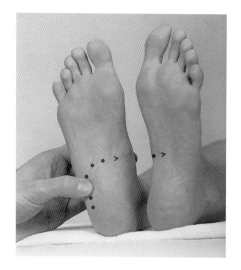

Combination of Simultaneous and One-Sided Massages

■ First massage both feet simultaneously as described above.

■ Then cover the left foot.

■ Position the thumb on the outer point of the right foot where the heel begins. Work along the edge of the foot and go up slightly until you

reach the upper margin of region 4. Traverse via the sole of the foot to the inner edge.

■ When you get there, cover the right foot and uncover the left one.

■ Continue at the same height on the right inner edge of the left foot and massage up to the outer edge. Continue to work in a crescent downward, back toward the inner edge. Here you will conclude with a few thumb pressure points.

Zones That Are Influenced by This Massage

Small Intestine and Colon

According to Fitzgerald, the fourth region encompasses the abdomen area, including the small intestine and colon.

The small intestine is very long, well over several feet (meters) and, thus, offers more than enough space to "tackle." Its reflex zones can be massaged firmly across the entire width of the soles of the feet.

▷
Left:
Upper margin of region 4 on the left foot. Massage with the left thumb.

Right:
Massage from the outer edge of the left foot downward in a crescent and toward the reflex point on the inner edge of the heel. Here, work with the right thumb.

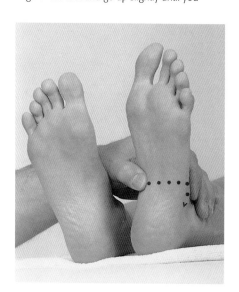

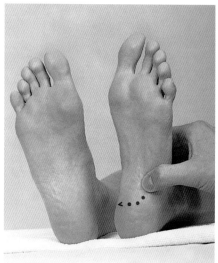

With intestinal inflammations (e.g., stomach flu, diarrhea, flatulence) only gentle pressure, stroking, and holding are recommended.

Lying on the right side of the body, the colon follows the small intestine. It begins as a rising branch, traverses the abdomen area, descends on the left side and flows into the intestine's final portion, the rectum, and into the anus. Generally, due to the overlapping of the small intestine and colon zones, the colon is always massaged when you are treating the reflex zones of the small intestine.

Both metaphorically and literally, we find lots of things to be "hard to digest." If you need to, massage the zone of the colon in addition to that of the small intestine either gently or with a little more force. Follow your intuition!

If you lose sight of the reflex zones of the colon because of the continuous change in direction, a glance at your own belly or that of your partner helps. Imagine how the colon runs and, corresponding to it, the reflexology runs.

If you have a disposition to flatulence, hard stool, or problems with hemorrhoids, massage the reflex zone of the anus on the inner foot with gentle pressure several times. Remain for a moment with the thumb positioned in a circling movement.

Do you recall that the reflex zone of the bladder lies right above this zone (see p. 66)? The bladder and the anus are only slightly separate in nature, so the reflex zones lay close to one another.

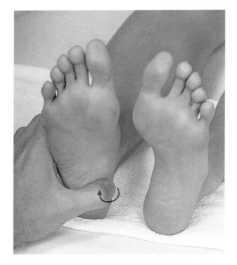

The region of the anus can be massaged on both right and left and can be supported with a slight rotation.

A healthy intestine contributes a great deal to one's general well-being. Therefore, always carefully massage the reflex zones of the intestine!

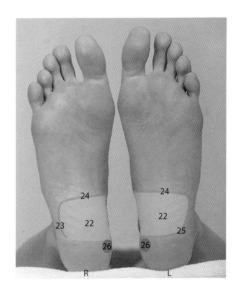

Massaged reflex zones in region 4:
22 Small intestine
23 Ascending colon
24 Traverse colon
25 Descending colon
26 Anus

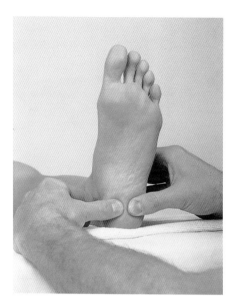

Reflexology of the heel.

Region 5

The Heel

The massage of the heel can be performed either consecutively or simultaneously.

- It is handled the same way as the massage of the reflex zones of the small intestine (see pp. 67–69).
- In addition, the work rhythm with this massage is continued via the body up to the head.

The Inner and Outer Ankles

The following area must be massaged on each foot separately.

- On both the right and left foot, massage the inner and outer edges of the foot below the ankles. As you touch with the pads of your fingers, you will feel that one spot is strikingly soft and sensitive on the inside. For practice, find this spot on your own foot first.
- Massage first the inside and then the outside, using either the thumb or the index and middle finger. One finger alone feels too "pointed." Make sure that the foot is well supported. You will find that it is possible to massage both inside and outside simultaneously.

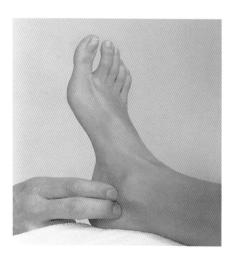
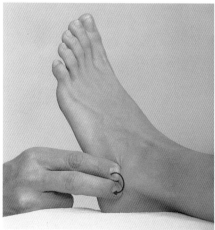

Left: Massage below the inner ankle with the index and middle fingers.

Right: Rotating massage below the outer ankle with both fingers.

■ For this, position your index and middle fingers right and left.

■ Massage three to four times from bottom to top. It feels very good to lay the fingers on the spot and rotate them (ill. p. 70 bottom right) or to stroke with the pads of your fingers around the ankle in a circular movement (ill. top right).

■ Afterward, the fingers of the right and left hand massage toward one another by way of the dorsum of the foot. Position your middle and/or index finger on the inside and the outside respectively.

■ Now move along below the ankle using of a pressure point massage (ill. bottom). Let your fingers run a little bit past one another on the dorsum of the foot; think of this as the "zipper principle." If the massaging fingers stop in front of one another, the person massaged may get the feeling that there is a "gap" in the massage.

As a final touch, you can perform a holding touch.

■ As you massage, work with both hands; place one palm on the zone between the inner ankle and the heel, and the other correspondingly on the reflex zone between the outer ankle and heel. You may even experience a cozy warmth arising from under your hands.

■ Imagine that you are shaping your hands in a protective fashion like an imaginary roof and form a small hollow with your palms.

■ For one or two breaths, hold your hands on the same spot before you remove them slowly and cautiously.

■ After you have covered the massaged foot, turn your attention to the other foot, and work your way through the respective reflex zones.

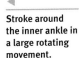
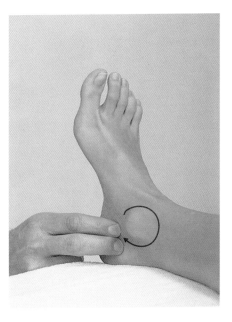

Stroke around the inner ankle in a large rotating movement.

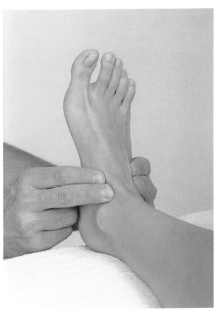

The fingers of the right and left hand work from outside to inside toward one another.

Zones That Are Influenced by This Massage

Pelvis and Pelvic Floor

The pelvis and pelvic floor regions are addressed in the area of the heel. A firm pelvis ensures a stable posture, both on the physical and the mental levels. Massaging the heel to treat the region of the pelvis reflex zones stabilizes us in both senses!

In both Taoist tradition and Indian chakra teaching, the stabilizing of the entire human being is centered upon the important area of the pelvis. In Hatha Yoga, Tai Chi, as well as Qigong, consciousness and breathing focus upon this center of the body. It is often considered the center of origin, the center for power, energy, and tranquility.

The straight sitting position, which might feel uncomfortable, is actually a posture resulting from a straightened pelvis. The shoulders hang loosely at the side, and the lungs, inner organs, and intestines have space to unfold, leading to better breathing and a good digestion. Thus, in this context, you should pay attention to the double meaning of what it means to be a "straight up" kind of a person.

As you can see, you should always include the heels in your massage. As a reflex zone, it stands for stability, and, as part of the foot, it acts as its concluding part.

▶

Massage reflex zones on the inner foot in region 5:
27 Pelvic floor
28 Uterus/ prostate
30 Fallopian tube/ spermatic duct/lymph in the groin area

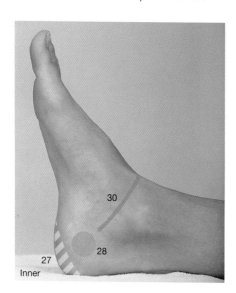

▶

Massage reflex zones on the outer foot in region 5:
27 Pelvic floor
29 Ovary/penis/ testicles
30 Fallopian tube/spermatic duct/lymph in the groin area

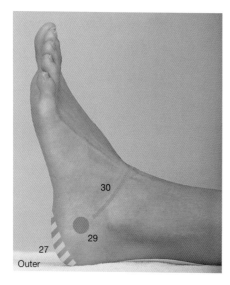

Uterus, Ovaries, Fallopian Tube/ Testicles, Prostate, Spermatic Duct, and Lymph Nodes of the Groin

Take a look once again at the zone chart or at the form analogy in the foot. If you transfer the areas of the reflex zones just discussed to the illustrations, you will arrive at the point where the reproductive organs are located.

The uterus is located in the middle of the pelvis. Hence, you massage the respective reflex zone on the inner edge of both the right and the left foot (zone 1 according to Fitzgerald). This holds true for the prostate as well.

The ovaries are positioned on the outer right and left in the pelvis, just above the uterus. The massage for the right ovary happens on the right, that of the left ovary on the left outer foot. The reflex zones of the testicles are likewise massaged on the outer edge of the foot. The connecting line between the inner and outer sides of the foot, which you have massaged with the pads of your fingers via the dorsum, corresponds to the fallopian tube or spermatic ducts. The fallopian tubes run from the ovaries toward the uterus, and the spermatic ducts from the testicles past the prostate toward the penis. The lymph nodes of the groin area stretch across on the level of the ovaries. Correspondingly, the reflex zone of the lymph nodes is stimulated with the massage via the dorsum of the foot, supporting lymph flow. This is recommended for people who have problems with the lymphatic system, people suffering from allergies, and people who experience a general lack of drive.

Holding can be very pleasant in the area of the reflex zone for the uterus or prostate. Both on the physical level and as a reflex zone, this area is very sensitive, so the massage should be carried out with great respect.

In times of significant physical change (puberty, first menstruation, voice change, menopause), the treatment in the area of the heel as well as the inner and outer ankle is very useful.

Wrapping Up the Massage—The Farewell

Your Posture

■ Are you satisfied when it comes to your own sitting position? If not, take the time necessary to arrange yourself before wrapping up your foot reflexology.
■ Be sure that you remain in contact with your partner's feet by way of a loosely positioned hand.

The Final Stroke

■ Conclude the massage with one of the stroking techniques listed in the chapter "Grips and Techniques That You Should Be Familiar With" (beginning on p. 34).

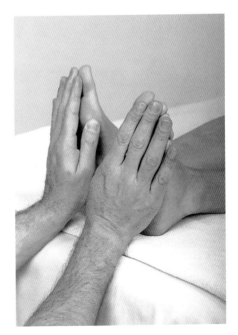

◀

The holding of the hands against the soles of the feet—a very pleasant ending to the foot reflexology.

■ There are several viable alternatives to use here: the energy stroke, holding the hands against the soles of the feet, gently pulling the feet toward you in order to stretch the spine, or massaging the feet with the knuckles.

■ Finally, carefully cover the feet. It feels very pleasant when you "snuggle" the blanket around the foot. In this way, your partner gets the feeling of caring and security.

The Farewell

■ Place both hands loosely on the knees and move with an uninterrupted stroking and slight pressure along the shin bones down to and off the ends of the feet.

■ Repeat this farewell gesture twice more.

■ Now you can conclude the entire massage with a brief pressure of both hands on the outer sides of the feet—think of it as the equivalent to shaking hands.

The Significance of This Wrapping-Up Ritual

If possible, you should adhere to the suggested farewell or to any other that you have chosen. The important point is that the massage ends in a recognizable ritual for both people involved.

Each session of foot reflexology needs a clear beginning and a clear end.

▶
The farewell ritual at the end of the foot reflexology is as important as the establishing of contact at the beginning.

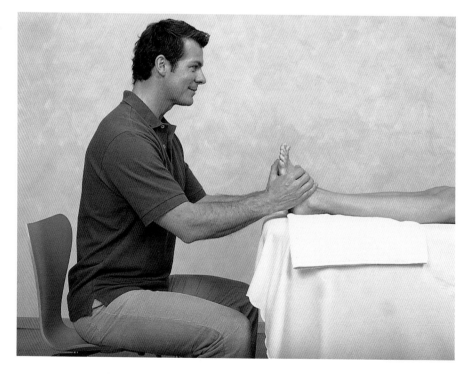

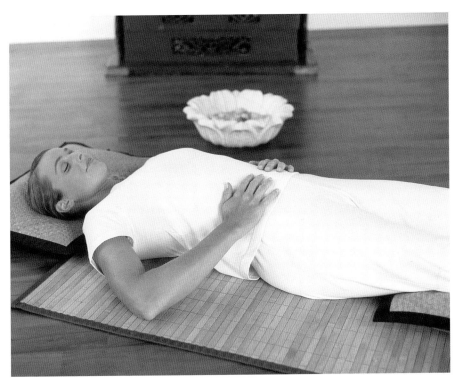

During the after-rest, the stimuli experienced during the massage fully unfold in the body.

The After-Rest

You should tell your partner prior to the massage that the after-rest is an important part of the treatment. The calming yet stimulating effect of foot reflexology is thus allowed to both linger and taper off.

The after-rest should last about 10 minutes.

The stimuli activated during the course of a foot reflexology continue to work in the body both after the massage and between the massages, and thus, the massage has an effect that lasts well beyond the actual treatment time.

"Brushing Off" After the Massage

If your partner feels slightly dazed following a foot reflexology treatment, you may "brush him off" a little while he is standing.

The brushing off has a refreshing and vitalizing effect.

■ For this, place yourself in front of your partner. Similar to the security frisking of the arms and legs at the airport, tap the person opposite you from top to bottom. With energy, begin by tapping two or three times along the arms, then down the torso, and finally all the way down the legs.

Special Foot Reflexologies

Self-Massage

In principle, self-massage is carried out in the same way as partner massage.

- Find a suitable position, on the bed, for example, or on a sofa.
- Bend your leg in an acute angle at the knee and pull the foot toward you. Place your foot either onto the other leg or next to it.
- You may also sit on a chair and rest your foot on another chair.
- Try out various positions to see which serves you best for the longest time, but you should change positions as soon as you notice that it becomes uncomfortable.

Procedure

- The self-massage follows the same suggested pattern of the two-person massage: Be sure that you work from top to bottom and from outside to inside even if you cannot always stick to the typical two-person ordering principles of a reflexology treatment, such as the direction of the massage or "thumb moves forward."

▇ **Your own comfort comes first.**

- When performing your massage, alternate between using the right and left thumbs. Also, you may use your index and middle fingers.
- As usual, the key is to try variations in order to find out how you can easily reach the necessary points.
- Always be attentive to your working speed and pressure intensity. Frequently one works too quickly during a self-massage.

▇ **Carry out all applications with care and attentiveness, just as you would in a partnered massage.**

Starting a Self-Massage

Indulge in a warm footbath before your foot reflexology treatment.

▼

Begin your self-massage with an energy stroke (see p. 78).

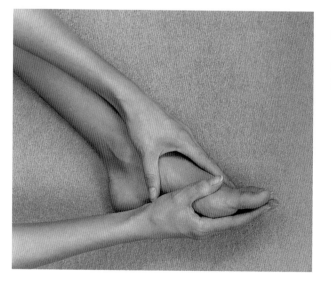

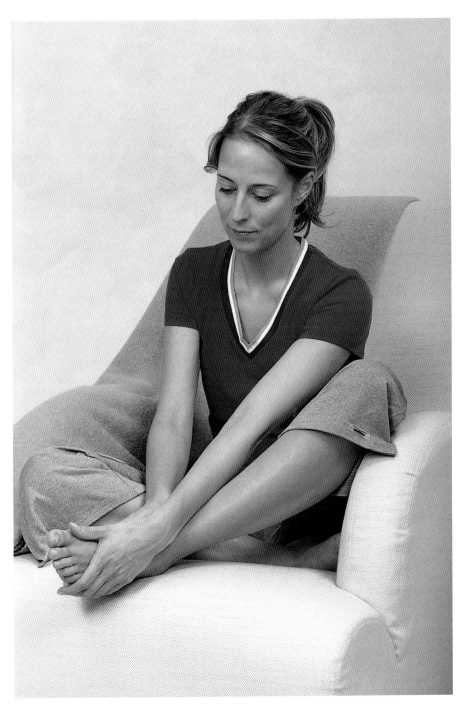

It is particularly important for the self-massage that you are seated very comfortably and can easily reach the foot to be massaged.

The Energy Stroke

■ Start with a modified type of the energy stroke (see p. 34) by moving with one hand from the toes across the sole of the foot to the heel, and, by stroking with the other hand in the opposite direction from the ankle joint across the dorsum of the foot back to the toes.

■ You can carry out this type of massage with both hands simultaneously or consecutively by first gliding with one hand across the sole and then with the other hand across the dorsum.

Other Stroking Techniques and Holding Positions

■ Stroking techniques and holding positions can be performed at the beginning of your massage, between individual regions, and at the end of the treatment (see pp. 34 and 38).

■ Give free rein to your hands when massaging. Most of the time, you will intuitively know which hold or stroke does you the most good.

With self-massage, stroking techniques and holding positions should be simple and effective. Sense how much warmth and tranquility can flow from your hands!

Region 1

■ As usual, start with the reflex zone of the spine; then massage each foot in succession from the toes downward, along the inner edge.

■ Massage along the edge of the bone, not on the bone!

▶
Left:
Holding and the energy stroke with the self-massage.

Right:
Self-massage of the spine reflex zone.

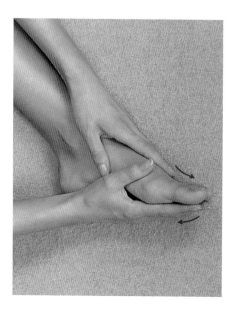
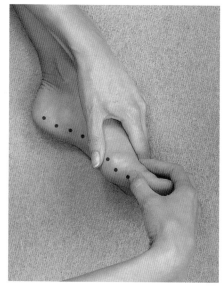

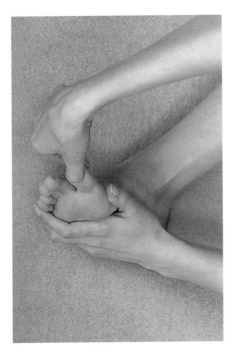

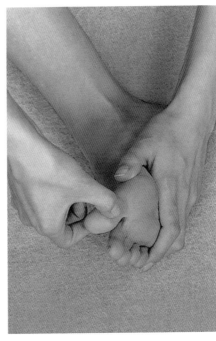

◄

Left:
Self-massage of toes.

Right:
Turning the toes with the self-massage. Be sure to grab the toe safely by its basal joint, with the additional support of the middle finger if necessary.

■ Repeat the treatment of the spine reflex zone. If you find painful spots, you should work them more than once. Always be mindful of your work rhythm.

■ After addressing the reflex zone of the spine, the toes, as the reflex zones of the head region, come next. Starting with the big toe, turn each individual toe at the basal joint (see p. 51).

■ Next massage either the big toe only or all the toes consecutively.

■ The "shoulder massage" is carried out the same as it is with the partnered massage: Massage with both thumbs from outside to inside, moving toward one another on the sole of the foot right below the toes.

Picture in your mind how you are treating your shoulders.

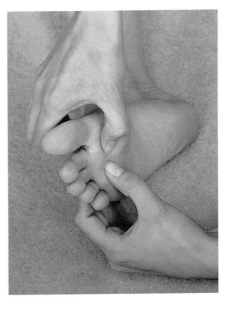

◄

Self-massage of the shoulder reflex zone.

▶

Reflex zones of the lungs and the bronchia for the self-massage.

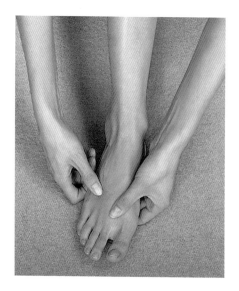

Region 2

Now address the zones of the lungs and bronchia on the dorsum of the foot. You can easily reach them with self-massage by working the space between the metatarsal bones—differing from the partnered massage—as you move away from your body and toward the toes.

■ For this, place your foot on a surface. With the left foot, use the right thumb for the first and second spaces between the metatarsals and the left thumb for the third and fourth spaces. Proceed correspondingly on the right foot: The left thumb for the two inner spaces, and right thumb for the two outer spaces.

▶

The liver reflex zone on the right foot can also be treated with both thumbs even with the self-massage.

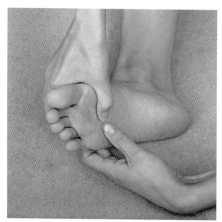

Region 3

■ One leg is bent, and the other foot rests on its outer edge. Use whichever thumb can comfortably reach each reflex zone and alternate correspondingly.

■ Massage consecutively the reflex zones of the thyroid, heart, stomach, liver (on the right foot), spleen (on the left foot), pancreas, solar plexus, kidneys, and bladder. You can treat the zone of the liver with both thumbs at the same time by having the right and the left thumb work toward one another, just as it is done in the partnered massage.

■ Massage the reflex zones of the third region first on one foot and then on the other. If your seating position becomes uncomfortable before the massage of the entire region is completed, simply change positions as needed.

▶

Reflex zone of the solar plexus for the self-massage.

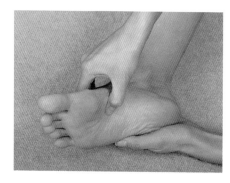

If, as you start your self-massage experience, you find that your treatment of all the zones takes too long, that your position feels odd, or that your time is too short, you will have to choose which points to treat: In region 3, treat the zones for the heart, liver, spleen, solar plexus, and kidneys, without addressing the urethra and the bladder.

Region 4

The reflex points of the intestine are well suited for treatment by a self-massage.

■ Massage the right foot with the right hand, and the left foot with the left hand. The thumbs work horizontally from inside to outside. If you can pull your foot closely enough to your body, so that it rests flatly in front of you, you can also work with both thumbs simultaneously toward one another.

■ Although the reflex zone of the colon can often be neglected with the self-massage, you can address it together with the zones of the small intestine.

Region 5

■ Massage the reflex zones of the pelvic floor on the heel, as well as the zones of the small intestine.

■ In addition, you can work in vertical lines with the left thumb on the right heel, again from inside to outside. The right thumb massages the left foot. Combining the three massage types is possible.

■ For treating the genital area, you are best off placing the foot on a surface. In this way, the uterus/prostate can be easily treated from the inside and the ovaries/testicles from the outside. Just as it is with the partnered massage, use your index and middle fingers, positioned on the right and left, slightly toward the back, and just below the ankle.

■ Massage two or three times before moving on in the direction of the dorsum. Here your fingers will come to a rest, separate from the fingers of the other hand.

■ Repeat this "stroll" along the ovary and lymph node reflex zones.

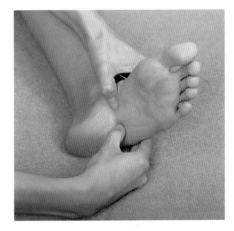

Reflex zone of the intestine with self-massage.

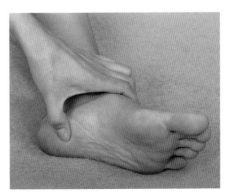

Self-massage of the pelvic reflex zone is possible both horizontally and vertically.

▶

Left:
Self-massage of the reflex zone of the uterus.

Right:
A calm and concentrated hold of the sensitive region of the uterus reflex zone.

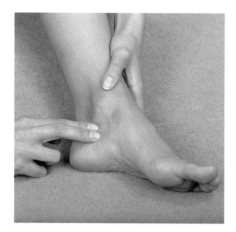

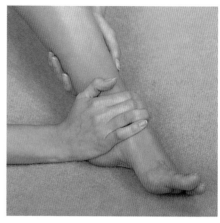

■ Finally, hold your palm on the zone of the uterus/prostate. For this, the foot should again be resting sideways.

■ Look at this sensitive area with new eyes thanks to the self-massage. Do you feel a sense of warmth or tranquility when your hand rests calmly on this reflex zone?

Wrapping Up Your Self-Massage

Wrap up your massage by holding the palms of your hands against the entire sole of the foot.

■ The right hand should lie under the left sole of the foot, while the left hand holds the dorsum.

■ With your hands, establish contact with your feet, and then build up a little pressure, comparable to a friendly handshake. This is precisely the attitude to bring into the conclusion of your self-massage.

■ Proceed with your right foot in the same fashion, only reversed.

■ For the beginning and the end of your self-massage, get into the habit of a specific ritual. This will give you a sense of security. Therefore, choose specific stroke movements and holding techniques that you will perform each time.

■ Spoil your feet after successful reflexology with a nice lotion or a fortifying cream.

▶

Wrapping up the self-massage with a warming, holding technique.

Brief Programs

Alleviating Stress

Stress—everyone knows it and feels its effects. While positive stress spurs our spirit of vitality, negative stress can cause afflictions of anxiety attacks, shallow breathing, racing heart, harassment, or digestive problems. Reflexology, partnered- or self-massage, can alleviate this pressure.

With this kind of massage, though, it is extremely important that you, as the person carrying out the massage, be well-balanced. Pay attention to your posture and breathing, ensuring that you have a calm and concentrated work ethic (see pp. 14 and 15, "Zone Charts," for the individual reflex zones).

■ Start with stroking movements, holding, and energy strokes (see p. 34).
■ You may either rotate all of the toes or only the big toe.
■ Massage the reflex zones of the pituitary and thyroid glands.
■ Change to the dorsum of the foot, and work the reflex zones of the lungs followed by some "ventilating."
■ Massage—again on the sole of the foot—the zones of the heart, liver, spleen, kidneys, and solar plexus. Heart, kidney, and solar plexus zones can be treated simultaneously on both feet. Massage the liver reflex zone with the left thumb on the right foot, while the right hand loosely reaches around the left foot. With the subsequent massage of the spleen reflex zone, you will proceed in reverse.
■ Then treat the reflex zone of the intestine in a calm rhythm on both sides.

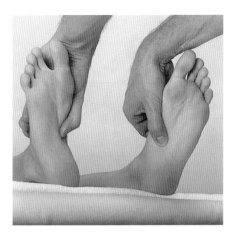

The hold for the solar plexus zone can be performed with each anti-stress massage.

■ The massage of both heels ends the anti-stress treatment and gives support.
■ "Contact to the ground" is important since the "grounding" is often the aspect most missing with stress.
■ Conclude the treatment by holding your hands against the soles of the feet.
■ As a farewell, stroke down the lower legs starting from the knees with gentle movements.

> For a couple of minutes before going to bed, massage the reflex zones of the spine, pituitary gland, heart, liver, solar plexus, and intestine. This will give you a great send-off for a refreshing night's sleep.

Fighting Fatigue, More Energy!

With this brief program, the reflex zones of the pituitary gland, thyroid gland, heart, liver, spleen, kidneys, solar plexus, and the pelvis are massaged (see p. 14).
■ Work with enthusiasm on both feet simultaneously.

▶
The energy point is held on both feet simultaneously.

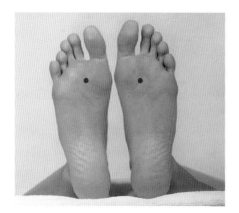

▪ Finally, you can hold the energy point on each foot simultaneously: With slight pressure, place your thumb centered in the ball of the foot. A pulsating feeling of warmth may arise. Concentrate on being calm and taking deep breaths. Check your body posture. Slowly relax the fingers when you or your partner has the feeling that it is enough. This is often the case after about 10 seconds.

■ Massage can release untapped energies and, in this way, lead to refreshing feelings of inner satisfaction. In the same way, it can help the person massaged to indulge in satisfying a need for tranquility.

Easing Tensions in the Neck, Shoulders, and Back

▪ With this treatment, the reflex zones of the spine, head (on the big toe on all four sides), and the area of the shoulder are attentively worked on.
▪ On the dorsum of the foot, shift to the zones of the lungs and bronchia.

▪ Back on the sole of the foot, work on the zones of the remaining regions. Here, you can introduce some variety. Be sure, though, to always include the reflex zones of the solar plexus and intestine. Experiment and alternate. Pay attention to how your partner reacts throughout the course of the massage, and "listen" to your fingers in case they want to wander to certain zones.
▪ Complementary to the foot massage, you may stroke both arms to help "unburden" the shoulders and neck. This helps with tensions and can be done both to lead into and out of the massage treatment.
▪ Place your hands on both shoulders of your partner, staying aware of your own calm, deep breaths. Quite frequently, as pressure and tension in the shoulders ease up solely through your touch, they will lower a bit.
▪ Now, with pressure, stroke along the arms down beyond the hands; repeat this twice more. Calmly ask if the arms feel any different after the stroking than before; they may possibly feel long, heavy, or warm. This has a positive effect on the neck and shoulders.

■ Since a human being does not only consist of individual, isolated organs, and since illnesses or ailments can have many reasons, you should never only treat the zones assigned to the ailing organ with a series of brief massages.

Hand Reflexology

◀ ▼

General Information Regarding the Massage of Hands

Speaking from experience, massaging the hands is not quite as intense and deeply penetrating as massaging the feet. Nevertheless, treating the hand reflex zones can have a relaxing and health-promoting effect as well.

The advantage of the hands lies in the fact that they can obviously be reached very easily, making them very well suited even for a brief self-massage.

Zone Partitioning

Dr. Fitzgerald's zone partitioning can also be applied to hand reflexology (see p. 10). The hands, just like the feet, allow for the partitioning in twice-five vertical and three horizontal lines. The zones of the abdomen organs, however, are positioned more closely together with hand reflexology and closer to the inner edge.

Grips and Techniques That You Should Be Familiar With

Reflexology of the hands does not differ in terms of modalities, grip techniques, and stroking techniques from those of the feet. Activating and soothing thumb grips, the pinching technique, the working direction from top to bottom and from inside to outside, an even rhythmic speed, and appropriate pressure all correspond to what you have learned of the massage of the feet.

In addition, with hand reflexology, each individual zone is treated two to three times.

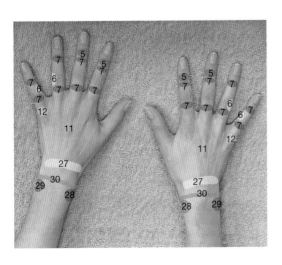

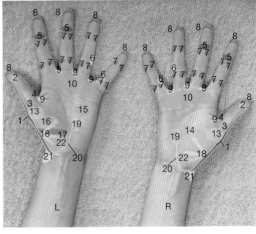

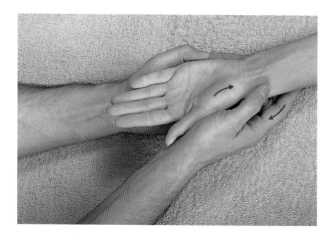

Stroking Techniques

Energy strokes can be performed on the hands in a modified version. You may have to stand up for this application though.

The energy stroke is carried out at the beginning and/or at the end of a massage.

■ For this, stroke along the palms, then up the arms until you reach the shoulders. At this point, circle the shoulders with generous pressure. Finally, move back down on the outer edge of the arm beyond the dorsum of the hands.

Preparations for the Massage

Placement

■ With this massage, your partner can sit on a bed, a chaise, an armchair, or any chair.

■ Just as you did during the massage of the feet, pay attention to your own straight sitting posture.

■ You can rest the massaged hand on your leg if this is comfortable for both of you, and feel free to use a pillow placed under the hand to improve the placement. Always see to it that there is sufficient distance—in the literal and the figurative sense—and experiment with various positions.

■ You should be able to massage from right and left. However, it is also possible to treat both hands from only one side if you are positioned comfortably.

Work Style

■ With the massage in regions 3 and 4, you can work on both hands simultaneously just as with the reflexology treatment of the feet.

■ With the hand massage, decide whether you want to completely massage each hand entirely and consecutively or to proceed region by region as was done with the feet.

■ **Try out both methods, and ask your partner which variation is more pleasant.**

Preparing the Hands

■ If the person to be massaged has very cold hands, take a well-preheated, damp towel and wrap each hand in it.

- Press the towel against the hands for a few moments, and then dry the hands well.
- You may also prepare a warm hand bath. This can be something as simple as a sink filled with warm water into which the forearms fit.
- If you have cold hands, you should definitely indulge in a hand bath before the treatment!

Hand reflexology is also very well suited for self-massage.

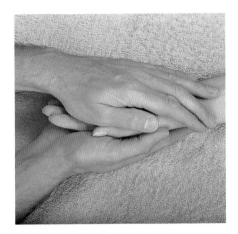

Holding and stroking the hands.

Order of the Hand Massage

The Greeting

- Establish contact with your partner, and begin the hand reflexology with holding and stroking.
- Take great care to notice your partner's hand, and, in doing so, concentrate fully on him or her.

Region 1

- The first part of the treatment is dedicated to the inner edge, from the tip of the thumb down to the beginning of the wrist.
- Use the pinching technique to massage the thumb and the remaining fingers consecutively. Begin just below the nail and end above the basal joint.

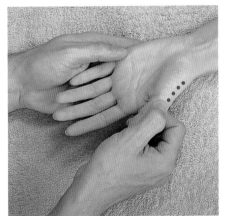

Reflexology on the outer side of the thumb.

Reflexology of the fingers.

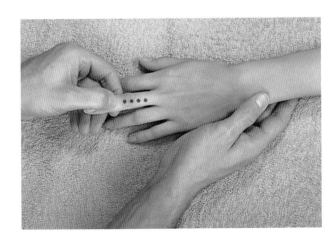

▶ ▼

Top:
Stroking the area between the fingers.

Middle:
The thumbs work across the entire width of the hand toward one another.

Bottom left:
Reflex zones of region 1:
 1 **Spine**
 2 **Pituitary gland**
 3 **Thyroid gland**
 4 **Palatal tonsils**
 5 **Eyes**
 6 **Ears**
 7 **Teeth**
 8 **Sinuses**
 9 **Lymph in the head region**
10 **Shoulder region**

Bottom right:
Reflex zones of region 2:
11 **Lungs**
12 **Shoulder joint/upper arm**

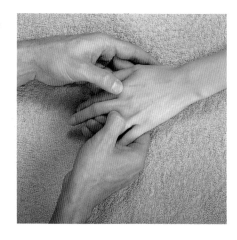

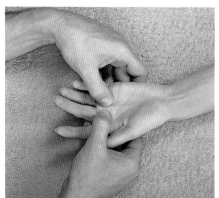

■ Massage with each finger on its upper and lower sides and—if you want—inner and outer sides.

■ Next, you should stroke the skin in all the areas between the fingers.

■ Now give your attention to the zone located in the palm below the fingers. Here, let your two fingers work from the outside to the inside and toward one another.

Zones That Are Influenced by This Massage

When massaging region 1, consecutively work the reflex zones of the spine and the entire area of the head through the thyroid gland, eyes, ears, and the teeth zones. You should also address the zones of the lymph region of the head and shoulder areas.

Stroking the areas between the fingers in terms of the lymphatic defense reflex area may feel slightly painful to a person with a weak immune system or a cold.

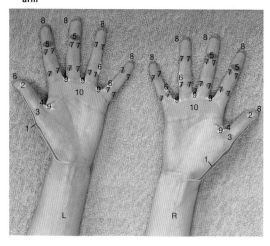

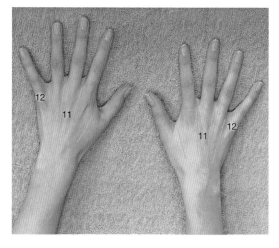

Region 2

Continue the massage on the dorsum of the hand.

■ Begin with the space between thumb and the index finger and, with the thumb grip, move downward until you can feel the beginning of the carpal bones. Proceed accordingly with the spaces between each of the other fingers.

■ Moving the carpal bones against each other wraps up the treatment for region 2. Support the hand from below with the ball of one hand, and, from above, place the tips of the fingers of the other hand in two adjacent spaces each. Move your hands in opposite directions from top to bottom and from bottom to top. Shift from one space to the next, just as you did with the foot reflexology (see p. 58).

Zones That Are Influenced by This Massage

When treating the dorsum of the hand, you are massaging the zones of the lungs and bronchia. This ventilation serves to "air" the lungs (see also p. 58).

> Frequent practice will change your movements from edgy and pushing to the more desirable wavy and flowing. Be patient with yourself!

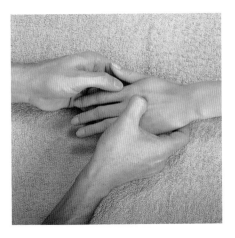

◀ Reflexology on the dorsum in the palpable spaces between the carpal bones.

Region 3

Immediately after this treatment of the hand's dorsum, follow with a massage of the ball of the hand and the palm.

■ With the thumb grip, work this entire area.

■ With the right hand, generously massage starting from the middle of the ball of the hand into the palm, toward the fingers, and up to just below the uppermost horizontal line of the hand.

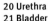

Reflex zones of region 3 in the palm:
13 Heart
14 Liver
15 Spleen
16 Stomach
17 Pancreas
18 Solar plexus
19 Kidneys
20 Urethra
21 Bladder

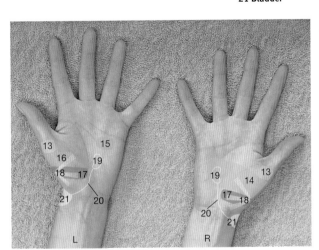

▶

Massaging the stomach reflex zone.

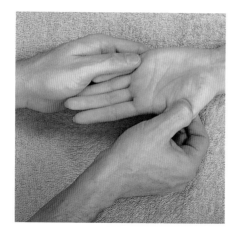

- On the left side, the massage is carried out from the middle of the ball only up to the second metacarpal bone below the index finger.
- Place your thumb on the center of the palm line that runs from the inner palm edge in a crescent toward the wrist. Massage here, and then move with the familiar pressure grips diagonally down and inward to the point where the hand meets the forearm. There is a reflex zone here that you will also massage.
- Now place your thumb in the middle of the ball. This is a sensitive area which, when stimulated, radiates outward.
- In this zone, you can try to work on both hands simultaneously.

Zones That Are Influenced by This Massage

On the right side, you will treat the zones of the heart, liver, kidney, and solar plexus; on the left side, you will work on the zones of the heart, stomach, spleen, kidney, and solar plexus.

▶

Massaging the kidney reflex zone.

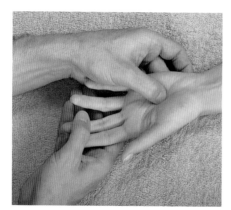

Region 4

All that remains to be massaged is the lower area of the palm up to the joint, the region of the carpal bones.

- You can work with one thumb from inside to outside or with both thumbs toward one another. With practice and good placement, it is also possible to use one thumb on each hand and thus massage simultaneously.

▶

Massaging the reflex zone of the urethra and bladder.

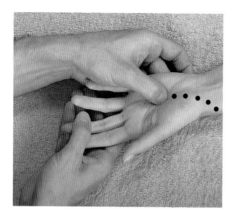

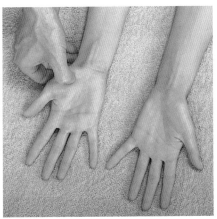

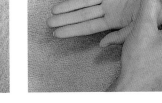

◀ ▼

Left:
Reflexology of the solar plexus.

Right:
Reflex zones of the small intestine.

Bottom left:
Reflex zones of region 4:
22 Small intestine
23 Ascending colon
24 Horizontal colon
25 Descending colon
26 Anus

Bottom right:
Reflex zones of region 5:
27 Pelvic floor
28 Uterus/ prostate
29 Ovary/ penis/ testicles
30 Fallopian tube/sper- matic duct/ lymph in the groin

Zones That Are Influenced by This Massage

The reflex zones worked in region 4 belong to the small intestine. If you are looking to support the intestines' functioning, it works best to massage these zones rhythmically on both sides.

If, in addition, you wish to stimulate the colon zone, begin on the right hand in the middle of the wrist. Move upward via the carpal bones, and turn right and slightly downward via the ball to the inner edge. Continue to the respective spot on the left hand where you then massage horizontally toward the outside. From the height of the index and small finger onward, move downward in a crescent again toward the inner hand. The massage ends on the inner side of the wrist. Just as with the foot, you have followed the ascending, horizontal, and descending branches of the colon.

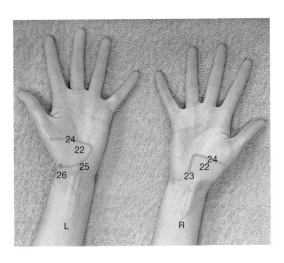

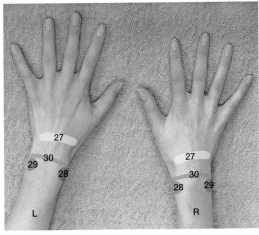

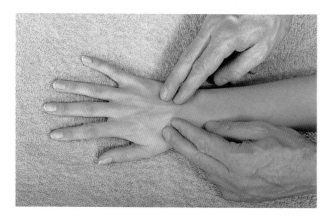

Reflexology of region 5: the lymph region in the pelvis and groin area.

Region 5

The next region is also located on the dorsum of the hand.

■ For your working grip, move your index and middle fingers of both hands horizontally across the wrist. In the same rhythm, let your fingers work toward one another from the outside to the inside.

Zones That Are Influenced by This Massage

With the massage below the carpal bones, you will activate the lymph region in the pelvis and

groin area. You will treat the genitals below the bladder at the inside and outside of the beginning of the carpal joint.

The Farewell

■ Wrap up the massage of the hand with stroking movements, holding, and/or an energy stroke.
■ As a farewell, lay your hands on the dorsum of your partner's hands, exert light pressure, and then slowly remove your hands.

> Both foot and hand reflexology can train the "perception" of your feeling.

Afterword

In this book, you have learned a lot about giving foot and hand reflexology treatments, about partnered massages and self-massages, about pressure points and potential reactions to a treatment. You may even have carried out a few massages already and have acquired some practical experience. What I would like to impart to you is the importance of the attention to your inner and outer "posture," for this creates greater sensitivity toward yourself. This is the best procedure for becoming more secure in the use of the massage: Trust your own intuition, and allow your hands to go their way. I wish you and your reflexology partners much joy with many massages!

A calm holding of the hand wraps up the massage.

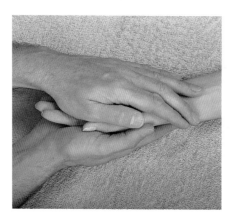

References

Resources

W.H. Fitzgerald and Edwin F. Bovers. *Zone Therapy or Relieving Pain at Home*. Columbus, Ohio: I. W. Long, 1917, and Los Angeles, California, 1918 Reprint of the edition appx. 1955, Imprint, Mokelumne Hill, Calif.: Health Research.

Eunice D. Ingham. *Stories the Feet Can Tell*, 2nd rev. ed. St. Petersburg, Fla.: Ingham Pub., June 1, 1984.

The collected work of *Stories the Feet Can Tell* (Volume I) and *Stories the Feet Have Told* (Volume II) can only be acquired in antique bookstores.

Association of Reflexologists
5 Fore Street
Taunton
Somerset, England
TA1 1HX
Tel: 0870 5673320 (Overseas: 01823 351010)
Email: info@aor.org.uk
www.aor.org.uk

International Council of Reflexologists
227 Dundas St. West
Paris, ON N3L 4H1
Canada
www.icr-reflexology.org

International Institute of Reflexology Inc.
5650 First Avenue North
P.O. Box 12642
St. Petersburg, FL 33733-2642
Tel: (727) 343-4811
Email: iir@tampabay.rr.com
www.reflexology-usa.net

National Practitioner Certification Board /American Reflexology Certification Board (ARCB)
P.O. Box 740879
Arvada, CO 80006-0879
Tel: 303 933 6921
Fax: 303 904 0460
Email: info@arcb.net
www.arcb.net

Reflexology Research
P.O. Box 35820
Albuquerque, NM 87176-5820
Tel: (505) 344-9392
Email: footcsc@swcp.com
www.reflexology-research.com

Reflexology Association of America
Administration Office
P.O. Box 26744
Columbus, OH 43226-0744
Tel: (740) 657-1695
www.reflexology-usa.org

Many states have individual state-based organizations. A Web search should turn up Web sites for organizations applicable to your own state.

Index

Author

Monika Schaefer is married and has three children. A nurse, she is also a registered German homeopath with an emphasis on foot reflexology. Monika has worked with various massage types for more than 20 years and intensively with reflexology for the past 10 years. Besides her practical work, she gives seminars on this topic and is an instructor for nursing staff, homeopaths, and laypersons.

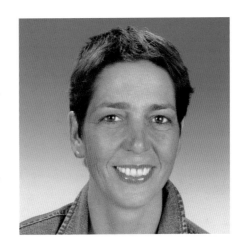

Acknowledgments

Many people have contributed to the making of this book, and I wish to warmly thank them: my foot reflexology teacher, Renate Roelofs-Perl from Cologne, who taught me so much. I also wish to express my gratitude to my husband for supporting all my activities and my children for being so patient. Likewise, I wish to thank Dr. Regina Degen for proofreading my work. And last, I wish to thank all the small and big people, who have entrusted their feet to me.

Credits

All photos Michael Reusse, except:
Getty Images, p. 9
Hart, Sammy p. 75
Parzinger, Dominik p. 44

Graphics: Jörg Maier, Munich